HEALTHC

Carbohydrate, Fat & Calorie Guide

Jane Stephenson, RD, CDE
Bridgett Wagener, RD

First Edition

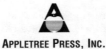

APPLETREE PRESS, INC.
Mankato, Minnesota

Appletree Press, Inc.
151 Good Counsel Drive Suite 125
Mankato, MN 56001

Phone: (507) 345-4848
Fax: (507) 345-3002
Website: www.appletree-press.com

The purpose of HealthCheques™: Carbohydrate, Fat & Calorie Guide is to supply authoritative data on the nutritional values of foods in a form for quick and easy reference. The information is not intended as a substitute for treatment prescribed by your physician. Please consult with your licensed health care professional before making any changes to your treatment plan.

CATALOGING-IN-PUBLICATION DATA

Stephenson, Jane, 1960-

HealthCheques™: Carbohydrate, Fat & Calorie Guide / authored by Jane Stephenson and Bridgett Wagener. Mankato, MN : Appletree Press, Inc., c1999.

112 p. : 15 cm.

Includes index.

Summary: This guide contains the best and most complete information available in a pocket counter. It was written as a reference to make healthy food choices. About 3,000 commonly (and not so commonly) eaten foods are grouped into easy-to-find categories and then listed alphabetically allowing the reader to track calories, carbohydrates, protein, fat, saturated fat, cholesterol, sodium and fiber. Charts and tables are included to determine daily nutrient goals.

ISBN 1-891011-02-2

1. Food—Composition—Tables. 2. Nutrition—Tables. 3. Food—Caloric content—tables. 4. Food—Cholesterol content—Tables. 5. Food—Fat content—Tables. 6. Food—Carbohydrate content—Tables. 7. Convenience foods—Composition—Tables I. Title II. Wagener, Bridgett, 1976-

613.28   99-90977

CIP

Editors: Linda Hachfeld and Gretchen Solting

Cover and Book Design: Douglas Allan Graphic Design

Printed in the United States of America

Sincere Thanks

We wish to thank our colleagues and publisher who contributed their time, expertise and inspiration in the development of HealthCheques™: Carbohydrate, Fat & Calorie Guide. We extend a special acknowledgment to Jackie Boucher, MS, RD, CDE, for her endless ideas, encouragement and assistance with the introduction of the book, and to Diane Bader for her expert editing skills and time spent organizing the book into user-friendly format.

We also thank our families and friends for their patience and understanding during the many hours of research involved in writing this book. Finally, we thank our HealthCheques™ customers who strive to achieve their nutrition and health goals each and every day.

Jane Stephenson, RD, CDE
Bridgett Wagener, RD
Authors

Contents

About This Book

HealthCheques™: Carbohydrate, Fat & Calorie Guide was written as a reference to help you make healthy food choices at home, on the run or in restaurants. It lists the calories, carbohydrate, protein, fat, saturated fat, cholesterol, sodium and fiber content of 3,000 foods and includes carbohydrate choices for persons with diabetes.

The foods in this guide are grouped into easy-to-find categories and then listed alphabetically from A to Z. Within each category you'll find subcategories. For example, under the category of Meats, the subcategories are Beef, Game, Lamb, Pork, Processed & Luncheon Meats and Specialty & Organ Meats. Serving sizes listed for individual foods within a category are consistent for easy comparison. Manufacturer's suggested servings are used in cases when serving sizes varied, such as in the Cereal section. Often two measures are given for foods that are available in more than one portion size; for example, Bagel, blueberry "1 (2 oz.)". Values listed inside parentheses such as Bagel, mini "2 (0.9 oz.)" refer to the value of each item; thus, each of the two mini bagels weigh 0.9 ounces.

Learn how to estimate your daily nutrient goals in three easy steps on page 96. To determine carbohydrate grams and choices by calorie level, please turn to page 97. Use the charts on page 98 and 99 to estimate the number of calories used during 30 minutes of various activities. In addition, you can track your blood lipid levels (Cholesterol, HDL, LDL and Triglycerides) on page 92.

This comprehensive guide is a terrific tool to help you stay healthy—keep it handy in your purse, pocket, desk drawer or glove compartment.

Abbreviations used in HealthCheques™

BBQ . . . . .barbecue		**n/a** . . . . . . .not available
con't. . . . . . .continued		**oz.** . . . . .ounce
fl. oz. . . . . . .fluid ounces		**pkg.** . . . . . . .package
frzn. . . . . . . .frozen		**pkt.** . . . . .packet
g . . . . .gram		**T.** . . . . .tablespoon
hmde. . . . . . .homemade		**tsp.** . . . . .teaspoon
in. . . . . .inch		**w/** . . . . .with
marg. . . . . . .margarine		**w/o** . . . . .without
mayo. . . . . . .mayonnaise		**/** . . . . .or
mg . . . . .milligram		*Example:*
		jam/jelly = jam "or" jelly

Nutrient values have been rounded to the nearest calorie, gram or milligram, with the exception of saturated fat values, which are rounded to the nearest 0.5 gram. Apparent inconsistencies may result from rounding off numbers, values may have been obtained from more than one source or samples of the same food, seasonal differences and slight variations among manufacturers.

Nutrient values change as products and recipes are reformulated and reanalyzed. Menu items listed may not be available at all restaurants and nutrient values for fast food restaurants are meant for general informational purposes only. Nutrient values are subject to change; values are current as of 1999. If the information you find on a label differs significantly from the data in this book, please use the label as your guide.

ALCOHOL

ITEM	AMOUNT	CALORIES	CARBOHYDRATE (g)	CARBOHYDRATE CHOICES	PROTEIN (g)	FAT (g)	SATURATED FAT (g)	CHOLESTEROL (mg)	SODIUM (mg)	FIBER (g)
ALCOHOL										
Beer										
light	12 fl. oz.	99	5	0	1	0	0.0	0	11	0
nonalcoholic	12 fl. oz.	78	14	1	1	0	0.0	0	9	0
regular	12 fl. oz.	146	13	1	1	0	0.0	0	18	0
Bloody Mary	8 fl. oz.	185	8	½	1	0	0.0	0	532	1
Bourbon & soda	4 fl. oz.	104	0	0	0	0	0.0	0	16	0
Brandy	1 fl. oz.	64	0	0	0	0	0.0	0	0	0
Brandy Alexander	4 fl. oz.	220	28	2	2	7	4.5	30	59	0
Champagne	4 fl. oz.	88	11	1	0	0	0.0	0	10	0
Cider, fermented	12 fl. oz.	160	11	1	0	0	0.0	0	10	0
Cordials/liqueurs, 54 proof	1 fl. oz.	106	13	1	0	0	0.0	0	2	0
Daiquiri	6 fl. oz.	336	12	1	0	0	0.0	0	9	0
Gin & tonic	8 fl. oz.	182	17	1	0	0	0.0	0	10	0
Gin/rum/vodka/whiskey										
80 proof	1 fl. oz.	64	0	0	0	0	0.0	0	0	0
86 proof	1 fl. oz.	70	0	0	0	0	0.0	0	0	0
90 proof	1 fl. oz.	73	0	0	0	0	0.0	0	0	0
100 proof	1 fl. oz.	82	0	0	0	0	0.0	0	0	0
Grasshopper	4 fl. oz.	229	39	2½	2	7	4.5	30	58	0
Irish coffee	8 fl. oz.	213	2	0	0	2	1.0	6	14	0
Irish cream	1 fl. oz.	137	7	½	1	6	3.5	14	33	0
Long Island iced tea	8 fl. oz.	216	16	1	0	0	0.0	0	11	0
Manhattan	4 fl. oz.	255	4	0	0	0	0.0	0	3	0
Margarita										
w/ salt	6 fl. oz.	370	23	1½	0	0	0.0	0	609	0
w/o salt	6 fl. oz.	370	23	1½	0	0	0.0	0	35	0
Martini	4 fl. oz.	252	0	0	0	0	0.0	0	3	0
Mudslide	4 fl. oz.	476	31	2	2	9	5.0	21	53	0
Piña colada	6 fl. oz.	296	38	2½	1	3	3.0	0	10	0
Rum & cola	8 fl. oz.	147	23	1½	0	0	0.0	0	29	0
Screwdriver	8 fl. oz.	199	21	1½	1	0	0.0	0	2	0
Tequila Sunrise	6 fl. oz.	206	16	1	1	0	0.0	0	7	0
Tom Collins	8 fl. oz.	130	3	0	0	0	0.0	0	40	0
Whiskey sour	4 fl. oz.	163	7	½	0	0	0.0	0	13	0
White Russian	4 fl. oz.	291	18	1	0	1	1.0	4	8	0
Wine, cooking										
Marsala	2 T.	35	2	0	0	0	0.0	0	190	0
red/white	2 T.	20	1	0	0	0	0.0	0	190	0
sherry	2 T.	29	0	0	0	0	0.0	0	180	0
Wine, table										
dessert, dry	4 fl. oz.	149	5	0	0	0	0.0	0	11	0

ALCOHOL

ITEM	AMOUNT	CALORIES	CARBOHYDRATE (g)	CARBOHYDRATE CHOICES	PROTEIN (g)	FAT (g)	SATURATED FAT (g)	CHOLESTEROL (mg)	SODIUM (mg)	FIBER (g)
Wine, table *(con't.)*										
dessert, sweet	4 fl. oz.	181	14	1	0	0	0.0	0	11	0
red/rosé	4 fl. oz.	85	2	0	0	0	0.0	0	6	0
sherry, dry	4 fl. oz.	82	2	0	0	0	0.0	0	9	0
spritzer	6 fl. oz.	105	2	0	0	0	0.0	0	14	0
white, dry/medium	4 fl. oz.	80	1	0	0	0	0.0	0	6	0
Wine cooler	12 fl. oz.	215	30	2	1	0	0.0	0	10	0

BEVERAGES

ITEM	AMOUNT	CALORIES	CARBOHYDRATE (g)	CARBOHYDRATE CHOICES	PROTEIN (g)	FAT (g)	SATURATED FAT (g)	CHOLESTEROL (mg)	SODIUM (mg)	FIBER (g)
Café latte										
w/ skim milk	8 fl. oz.	80	11	1	8	1	0.0	3	113	0
w/ whole milk	8 fl. oz.	140	11	1	7	7	5.0	30	107	0
Café mocha, w/ whipped cream										
w/ skim milk	8 fl. oz.	200	24	1½	9	11	6.0	40	110	0
w/ whole milk	8 fl. oz.	250	23	1½	9	16	10.0	55	105	0
Cappuccino										
w/ skim milk	8 fl. oz.	53	7	½	5	0	0.0	3	73	0
w/ water, mix	8 fl. oz.	90	18	1	1	1	0.0	0	65	0
w/ whole milk	8 fl. oz.	93	7	½	5	5	3.0	20	70	0
Capri Sun®	6.75 fl. oz.	100	27	2	0	0	0.0	0	20	0
Club soda/seltzer	8 fl. oz.	0	0	0	0	0	0.0	0	50	0
Coffee										
brewed/instant	6 fl. oz.	4	1	0	0	0	0.0	0	4	0
flavored mixes	6 fl. oz.	60	8	½	1	3	0.5	0	105	0
Crystal Light®	8 fl. oz.	5	0	0	0	0	0.0	0	0	0
Espresso	3 fl. oz.	8	1	0	0	0	0.0	0	12	0
Frappuccino®	9.5 fl. oz.	190	39	2½	6	3	2.0	12	110	0
Fruit punch	8 fl. oz.	117	30	2	0	0	0.0	0	55	0
Gatorade®/sports drink	8 fl. oz.	60	15	1	0	0	0.0	0	96	0
Hi-C®	8 fl. oz.	120	32	2	0	0	0.0	0	150	0
Hot cocoa, mix										
w/ 1% milk	8 fl. oz.	197	31	2	7	5	2.0	7	212	0
w/ water	8 fl. oz.	120	22	1½	1	3	1.0	0	120	0
w/ whole milk	8 fl. oz.	232	31	2	7	9	5.0	25	241	0
Kool-Aid®										
regular	8 fl. oz.	100	25	1½	0	0	0.0	0	20	0
sugar free	8 fl. oz.	5	0	0	0	0	0.0	0	5	0
Lemonade										
regular	8 fl. oz.	99	26	2	0	0	0.0	0	7	0
sugar free	8 fl. oz.	4	0	0	0	0	0.0	0	0	0
Quinine/tonic water	8 fl. oz.	83	21	1½	0	0	0.0	0	10	0
Soda, diet, most varieties	12 fl. oz.	0	0	0	0	0	0.0	0	35	0

BEVERAGES

ITEM	AMOUNT	CALORIES	CARBOHYDRATE (g)	CARBOHYDRATE CHOICES	PROTEIN (g)	FAT (g)	SATURATED FAT (g)	CHOLESTEROL (mg)	SODIUM (mg)	FIBER (g)
Soda, regular										
7 up®	12 fl. oz.	140	39	2½	0	0	0.0	0	75	0
Cherry Coke®	12 fl. oz.	150	42	3	3	0	0.0	0	45	0
Coca-Cola®	12 fl. oz.	140	39	2½	0	0	0.0	0	50	0
cream	12 fl. oz.	180	46	3	0	0	0.0	0	45	0
Dr. Pepper®	12 fl. oz.	150	40	2½	0	0	0.0	0	55	0
ginger ale	12 fl. oz.	140	36	2½	0	0	0.0	0	25	0
grape	12 fl. oz.	170	43	3	0	0	0.0	0	35	0
Mountain Dew®	12 fl. oz.	170	46	3	0	0	0.0	0	70	0
Orange Slice®	12 fl. oz.	170	46	3	0	0	0.0	0	55	0
Pepsi®	12 fl. oz.	150	41	3	0	0	0.0	0	35	0
root beer	12 fl. oz.	170	46	3	0	0	0.0	0	45	0
Ruby Red Squirt®	12 fl. oz.	180	47	3	0	0	0.0	0	23	0
Sprite®	12 fl. oz.	140	38	2½	0	0	0.0	0	70	0
Squirt®	12 fl. oz.	150	41	3	0	0	0.0	0	23	0
Surge®	12 fl. oz.	170	46	3	0	0	0.0	0	40	0
Sunny Delight®	8 fl. oz.	120	29	2	0	0	0.0	0	190	0
Tang®	8 fl. oz.	100	24	1½	0	0	0.0	0	0	0
Tea										
brewed/instant	6 fl. oz.	2	1	0	0	0	0.0	0	5	0
iced, diet	8 fl. oz.	5	0	0	0	0	0.0	0	5	0
iced, sweetened	8 fl. oz.	90	22	1½	0	0	0.0	0	0	0
Water, bottled	8 fl. oz.	0	0	0	0	0	0.0	0	2	0
Yoo-hoo®	8 fl. oz.	130	29	2	2	1	0.5	0	180	0

BREADS & BREAD PRODUCTS
Breads & Muffins

ITEM	AMOUNT	CALORIES	CARBOHYDRATE (g)	CARBOHYDRATE CHOICES	PROTEIN (g)	FAT (g)	SATURATED FAT (g)	CHOLESTEROL (mg)	SODIUM (mg)	FIBER (g)
Bagels										
blueberry										
medium	1 (2 oz.)	160	32	2	5	1	0.0	0	260	1
large	1 (3.7 oz.)	280	57	4	10	2	0.5	0	490	2
cinnamon raisin										
medium	1 (2 oz.)	160	32	2	5	1	0.0	0	240	1
large	1 (3.7 oz.)	280	59	4	10	2	0.5	0	490	3
egg										
medium	1 (2 oz.)	160	30	2	6	2	0.0	10	320	1
large	1 (3.7 oz.)	280	59	4	10	3	0.0	25	560	2
plain										
mini	2 (0.9 oz.)	140	28	2	5	1	0.0	0	260	1
medium	1 (2 oz.)	150	30	2	6	1	0.0	0	320	1
large	1 (3.7 oz.)	280	56	4	10	2	0.5	0	530	2
Bialys	1 medium	201	42	3	6	1	0.0	0	822	2

BREADS & BREAD PRODUCTS
Breads & Muffins

ITEM	AMOUNT	CALORIES	CARBOHYDRATE (g)	CARBOHYDRATE CHOICES	PROTEIN (g)	FAT (g)	SATURATED FAT (g)	CHOLESTEROL (mg)	SODIUM (mg)	FIBER (g)
Biscuits										
baking powder, can	1 (2 oz.)	200	25	1½	4	9	2.0	0	580	0
baking powder, hmde.	1 (1.4 oz.)	160	25	1½	4	5	1.0	0	460	1
buttermilk, can	1 (2 oz.)	190	24	1½	4	9	2.5	0	600	0
buttermilk, hmde.	1 (1.4 oz.)	170	24	1½	3	8	3.0	0	420	1
Breads										
Boston brown, can	1 slice	88	19	1	2	1	0.0	0	284	2
challah/egg	1 slice	115	19	1	4	2	0.5	20	197	1
cracked wheat	1 slice	74	14	1	2	1	0.5	0	153	2
French/Vienna	1 slice	69	13	1	2	1	0.0	0	152	1
fruit	1 slice	150	23	1½	2	6	1.5	22	109	1
garlic	1 (2 in.)	160	19	1	6	7	2.0	10	260	2
Irish soda	1 slice	174	34	2	4	3	0.5	11	239	2
Italian	1 slice	81	15	1	3	1	0.0	0	175	1
low protein	1 slice	90	19	1	0	2	0.0	1	7	2
multigrain	1 slice	100	18	1	4	2	0.0	0	160	2
oatmeal	1 slice	73	13	1	2	1	0.0	0	162	1
pita, white	1 (6 in.)	165	33	2	5	1	0.0	0	322	1
pita, whole wheat	1 (6 in.)	170	35	2	6	2	0.0	0	340	5
pumpernickel	1 slice	65	12	1	2	1	0.0	0	174	2
raisin	1 slice	71	14	1	2	1	0.0	0	101	1
rye	1 slice	83	15	1	3	1	0.0	0	211	2
sourdough	1 slice	69	13	1	2	1	0.0	0	152	1
wheatberry	1 slice	100	18	1	3	2	0.0	0	200	2
white	1 slice	65	12	1	2	1	0.0	0	130	0
white, light	1 slice	41	9	½	2	1	0.0	0	91	1
whole wheat	1 slice	69	13	1	3	1	0.0	0	150	2
whole wheat, light	1 slice	40	9	½	2	0	0.0	0	95	2
Breadsticks, soft	1 (2 oz.)	150	28	2	7	2	0.5	0	290	1
Cornbread	1 (2 oz.)	188	29	2	4	6	1.5	37	467	1
Croissants	1 (2 oz.)	231	26	2	5	12	6.5	38	424	1
English muffins										
plain	1 medium	134	26	2	4	1	0.0	0	264	2
raisin	1 medium	139	28	2	4	2	0.0	0	255	2
whole wheat	1 medium	127	26	2	5	1	0.0	0	218	3
Melba toast	4	78	15	1	2	1	0.0	0	166	1
Muffins										
banana nut	1 (2 oz.)	172	30	2	3	5	1.5	12	288	1
blueberry	1 (2 oz.)	158	27	2	3	4	1.0	17	255	1
blueberry, Sweet Rewards®	1 (2 oz.)	120	27	2	2	0	0.0	0	200	0
bran	1 (2 oz.)	163	24	1½	4	7	1.5	20	333	4
chocolate chip	1 (2 oz.)	190	27	2	4	8	3.0	25	186	1

BREADS & BREAD PRODUCTS
Breads & Muffins

ITEM	AMOUNT	CALORIES	CARBOHYDRATE (g)	CARBOHYDRATE CHOICES	PROTEIN (g)	FAT (g)	SATURATED FAT (g)	CHOLESTEROL (mg)	SODIUM (mg)	FIBER (g)
Muffins *(con't.)*										
corn	1 (2 oz.)	174	29	2	3	5	1.0	15	297	2
cranberry nut	1 (2 oz.)	164	25	1½	4	5	1.5	39	326	1
lemon poppy seed	1 (2 oz.)	215	34	2	4	8	2.0	24	263	1
pumpkin	1 (2 oz.)	181	34	2	3	4	1.0	26	154	1
Muffins, Dunkin' Donuts®										
banana, lowfat	1 (3.4 oz.)	240	54	3½	3	2	0.0	0	380	1
blueberry	1 (3.4 oz.)	310	51	3½	5	10	2.5	35	190	2
blueberry, lowfat	1 (3.4 oz.)	230	51	3½	3	2	0.0	0	370	1
chocolate chip	1 (3.4 oz.)	400	63	4	5	16	6.0	35	190	2
corn	1 (3.4 oz.)	350	51	3½	6	14	0.5	50	310	2
corn, lowfat	1 (3.4 oz.)	250	55	3½	4	2	0.0	0	460	1
honey raisin bran	1 (3.4 oz.)	330	57	4	5	10	0.0	15	360	4
Popovers	1 (2 oz.)	128	16	1	5	5	1.5	67	116	0
Rolls										
brown & serve	1 medium	84	14	1	2	2	0.5	0	146	1
crescent	1 medium	102	11	1	2	6	1.0	0	216	0
French	1 medium	105	19	1	3	2	0.0	0	231	1
hamburger	1 medium	123	22	1½	4	2	0.5	0	241	1
hard	1 medium	167	30	2	6	2	0.0	0	310	1
hot dog	1 medium	114	20	1	3	2	0.5	0	224	1
kaiser	1 medium	190	36	2½	6	3	1.0	0	340	2
rye	1 medium	81	15	1	3	1	0.0	0	253	2
sesame seed	1 medium	140	23	1½	5	3	1.5	0	240	1
sourdough	1 medium	131	25	1½	4	1	0.0	0	261	1
submarine	1 (8 in.)	230	50	3	9	2	0.5	0	500	2
whole wheat	1 medium	75	14	1	2	1	0.0	0	136	2
yeast	1 medium	90	17	1	2	2	0.5	0	130	0
Scones										
commercial	1 large	303	37	2½	8	13	4.0	104	498	1
homemade	1 medium	150	18	1	4	7	2.0	51	246	1
Bread Products										
Corn fritters	1 (2 oz.)	130	16	1	3	7	2.0	5	310	1
Crêpes	1 (3.5 oz.)	239	22	1½	9	12	4.0	163	274	1
Croutons	¼ cup	47	6	½	1	2	0.5	0	124	1
French toast										
frozen	1 slice	126	19	1	4	4	1.0	48	292	1
homemade	1 slice	149	16	1	5	7	2.0	75	311	1
Lefse	1 (2 oz.)	150	30	2	4	2	0.0	0	330	2
Pancakes										
blueberry, mix	2 (4 in.)	166	31	2	5	3	1.0	10	526	1
buttermilk, mix	2 (4 in.)	160	30	2	5	2	1.0	17	519	1

BREADS & BREAD PRODUCTS
Bread Products

ITEM	AMOUNT	CALORIES	CARBOHYDRATE (g)	CARBOHYDRATE CHOICES	PROTEIN (g)	FAT (g)	SATURATED FAT (g)	CHOLESTEROL (mg)	SODIUM (mg)	FIBER (g)
Pancakes *(con't.)*										
plain, frzn.	2 (4 in.)	165	31	2	4	2	0.5	6	366	1
plain, hmde.	2 (4 in.)	173	22	1½	5	7	1.5	45	334	1
plain, lowfat, frzn.	2 (4 in.)	100	20	1	3	1	0.0	0	353	1
whole wheat, mix	2 (4 in.)	112	15	1	4	4	1.0	36	288	1
Pizza crusts, Boboli®	1 (6 in.)	300	48	3	12	6	2.0	0	600	1
Pretzels, soft	1 large	340	72	5	10	1	0.0	0	900	3
Stuffing										
bread, hmde.	½ cup	195	26	2	4	8	1.5	0	535	2
cornbread, box	½ cup	179	22	1½	3	9	2.0	0	455	3
Stove Top®, box	½ cup	176	21	1½	5	9	5.0	21	632	3
Taco shells, hard	1 (5 in.)	62	8	½	1	3	0.5	0	49	1
Tortillas										
corn	1 (6 in.)	58	12	1	1	1	0.0	0	42	1
flour	1 (8 in.)	115	20	1	3	2	0.5	0	169	1
Waffles										
Belgian, mix	1 (3.6 oz.)	370	47	3	8	17	9.0	130	1020	1
blueberry, Eggo®, frzn.	1 (1.3 oz.)	100	15	1	3	4	1.0	10	210	1
homestyle, Eggo®, frzn.	1 (1.3 oz.)	95	15	1	3	4	1.0	10	220	1
plain, hmde.	1 (2.5 oz.)	218	25	1½	6	11	2.0	52	383	1
plain, lowfat, frzn.	1 (1.3 oz.)	80	16	1	3	1	0.0	0	270	1

CANDY

ITEM	AMOUNT	CALORIES	CARBOHYDRATE (g)	CARBOHYDRATE CHOICES	PROTEIN (g)	FAT (g)	SATURATED FAT (g)	CHOLESTEROL (mg)	SODIUM (mg)	FIBER (g)
Almonds										
candy-coated	10	154	22	1½	3	5	0.5	0	4	0
chocolate covered	10	190	27	2	2	10	5.0	5	90	0
Bridge mix	¼ cup	180	27	2	2	9	4.5	5	35	0
Butterfinger BB's®	¼ cup	200	29	2	2	8	5.0	0	85	0
Cadbury Eggs®, creme	1 (1.4 oz.)	170	29	2	1	6	4.0	0	25	0
Candy bars, average size										
100 Grand®	1 (1.5 oz.)	200	30	2	2	8	5.0	10	75	0
5th Avenue®	1 (2 oz.)	280	38	2½	5	12	4.5	0	95	1
Almond Joy®	1 (1.76 oz.)	240	29	2	2	13	8.0	0	70	2
Baby Ruth®	1 (2.1 oz.)	270	36	2½	4	13	7.0	0	130	2
Bit-o-Honey®	1 (1.7 oz.)	200	41	3	1	4	2.5	0	105	1
Butterfinger®	1 (2.1 oz.)	270	42	3	3	11	5.0	0	130	1
Caramello®	1 (1.6 oz.)	220	29	2	3	10	6.0	10	60	0
Chunky®	1 (1.4 oz.)	210	24	1½	3	11	6.0	5	20	1
Clark®	1 (1.75 oz.)	240	33	2	4	10	4.0	0	106	3
Heath Bar®	1 (1.4 oz.)	210	25	1½	1	13	6.0	10	150	0
Hershey's®, w/ almonds	1 (1.45 oz.)	230	20	1	5	14	7.0	5	35	1
Hershey's® milk chocolate	1 (1.55 oz.)	230	25	1½	3	13	9.0	10	40	1

CANDY

ITEM	AMOUNT	CALORIES	CARBOHYDRATE (g)	CARBOHYDRATE CHOICES	PROTEIN (g)	FAT (g)	SATURATED FAT (g)	CHOLESTEROL (mg)	SODIUM (mg)	FIBER (g)
Candy bars, average size *(con't.)*										
Kit Kat®	1 (1.5 oz.)	220	27	2	3	11	7.0	5	30	0
Krackle®	1 (1.45 oz.)	220	25	1½	3	12	7.0	10	55	1
Mars®	1 (1.76 oz.)	240	31	2	3	13	4.0	5	70	1
Milky Way®	1 (2.05 oz.)	270	41	3	2	10	5.0	5	95	1
Milky Way® lite	1 (1.57 oz.)	170	34	2	1	5	2.5	5	80	1
Mounds®	1 (1.9 oz.)	250	31	2	2	13	11.0	0	80	3
Mr. Goodbar®	1 (1.75 oz.)	270	25	1½	5	17	7.0	0	20	2
Nestle's Crunch®	1 (1.55 oz.)	230	29	2	2	12	7.0	10	65	0
Oh Henry!®	1 (1.8 oz.)	230	32	2	6	9	4.0	3	125	2
Pearson's® nut roll	1 (1.8 oz.)	240	27	2	8	11	2.0	0	170	2
Reese's Peanut Butter Cups®	2 (0.8 oz.)	250	25	1½	5	14	5.0	5	140	1
Skor®	1 (1.38 oz.)	206	21	1½	1	13	9.0	24	90	0
Snickers®	1 (2.07 oz.)	280	36	2½	4	14	5.0	10	150	1
Three Musketeers®	1 (2.13 oz.)	260	46	3	2	8	4.0	5	10	1
Twix®	1 (2 oz.)	280	37	2½	3	14	5.0	5	115	1
Candy corn	¼ cup	182	45	3	0	1	0.0	0	106	0
Caramels	5	160	31	2	2	4	1.0	5	100	0
Cherries, chocolate covered	2	150	29	2	0	4	2.0	0	10	0
Circus peanuts	6	150	38	2½	0	0	0.0	0	15	0
Cotton candy	2 oz.	220	57	4	0	0	0.0	0	0	0
Divinity, hmde.	2 (0.4 oz.)	77	10	½	0	0	0.0	0	10	0
Dots®	12	150	37	2½	0	0	0.0	0	20	0
Fondant	2 (0.5 oz.)	115	30	2	0	0	0.0	0	13	0
Fudge, hmde.										
chocolate, w/ nuts	1 oz.	121	21	1½	1	5	2.0	4	17	0
chocolate, w/o nuts	1 oz.	108	23	1½	0	2	1.0	4	18	0
vanilla, w/ nuts	1 oz.	118	21	1½	1	4	1.0	4	17	0
vanilla, w/o nuts	1 oz.	105	23	1½	0	2	1.0	5	19	0
Goobers®	¼ cup	220	21	1½	5	14	5.0	5	15	2
Good & Plenty®	35	140	35	2	1	0	0.0	0	85	0
Good 'n Fruity®	33	130	29	2	0	0	0.0	0	65	1
Gum, regular/sugar free	1 stick	10	2	0	0	0	0.0	0	0	0
Gumdrops	12	150	37	2½	0	0	0.0	0	20	0
Gummy bears	15	140	31	2	3	0	0.0	0	21	0
Hard candies										
regular	3 small	60	16	1	0	0	0.0	0	10	0
sugar free	3 small	36	10	½	0	0	0.0	0	0	0
Hershey's Hugs®	8	210	22	1½	3	12	6.0	10	35	0
Hershey's Kisses®	8	210	23	1½	3	12	8.0	10	35	1
Hot Tamales®	19	150	36	2½	0	0	0.0	0	15	0
Jelly beans	35 small	140	37	½	0	0	0.0	0	10	0

CANDY

ITEM	AMOUNT	CALORIES	CARBOHYDRATE (g)	CARBOHYDRATE CHOICES	PROTEIN (g)	FAT (g)	SATURATED FAT (g)	CHOLESTEROL (mg)	SODIUM (mg)	FIBER (g)
Jolly Rancher®	3	70	17	1	0	0	0.0	0	15	0
Junior® mints	16	160	34	2	0	3	2.0	0	5	0
Licorice, black/red	3 (8 in.)	120	27	2	1	0	0.0	0	85	0
Lifesavers®	2	20	5	0	0	0	0.0	0	0	0
Lollipops	1	22	6	½	0	0	0.0	0	2	0
M&M's®										
crispy	52	200	30	2	2	9	5.0	5	65	1
peanut	18	250	30	2	5	13	5.0	5	25	2
plain	52	240	34	2	2	10	6.0	5	30	1
Marshmallows	6 large	110	26	2	0	0	0.0	0	10	0
Mary Janes®	7	160	31	2	4	4	0.0	0	45	1
Mike and Ike®	19	150	36	2½	0	0	0.0	0	15	0
Milk Duds®	13	180	30	2	1	6	4.5	0	90	0
Mints										
breath	2	20	0	0	0	0	0.0	0	0	0
butter	6	51	12	1	0	0	0.0	0	21	0
Nips®, caramel	2	60	11	1	0	2	1.0	0	40	0
Orange slices	3	150	37	2½	0	0	0.0	0	15	0
Peanut brittle	½ cup	180	30	2	4	5	1.0	0	130	1
Peanuts, chocolate covered	¼ cup	193	18	1	5	12	5.5	3	15	2
Praline, hmde.	1 (1.4 oz.)	177	24	1½	1	9	0.5	0	24	1
Raisinets®	¼ cup	200	31	2	2	8	4.5	0	15	1
Raisins, yogurt covered	¼ cup	190	34	2	2	6	4.0	4	21	1
Red Hot Dollars®	10	140	34	2	0	0	0.0	0	0	0
Reese's Pieces®	50	190	22	1½	1	9	6.0	0	75	1
Rolo®	9	260	36	2½	3	11	6.0	10	110	0
Skittles®	¼ cup	170	37	2½	0	2	0.0	0	5	0
Starburst®	12	240	48	3	0	5	1.0	0	0	0
Sugar Babies®	32	190	43	3	0	2	0.0	0	75	0
Sugar Daddy®	1 (1.7 oz.)	200	43	3	1	3	0.5	0	100	0
Sweet Escapes Bars, Hershey's®										
caramel &										
peanut butter	1 (0.7 oz.)	70	12	1	1	3	1.0	0	75	0
caramel fudge	1 (0.7 oz.)	80	14	1	0	2	1.0	0	55	0
peanut butter	1 (0.7 oz.)	90	13	1	2	3	2.0	0	50	0
Taffy										
saltwater	5 small	140	32	2	1	2	1.0	0	80	0
Tangy Taffy®	1 (1.5 oz.)	170	35	2	0	4	3.5	0	20	0
Tootsie Pop®	1	50	12	1	0	0	0.0	0	10	0
Tootsie Roll®	6 small	160	33	2	0	3	0.5	0	40	1
Truffles, hmde.	2 (0.4 oz.)	117	11	1	1	8	4.5	12	17	1
Turtles	2 (0.6 oz.)	165	20	1	2	9	3.5	7	32	1

CANDY

ITEM	AMOUNT	CALORIES	CARBOHYDRATE (g)	CARBOHYDRATE CHOICES	PROTEIN (g)	FAT (g)	SATURATED FAT (g)	CHOLESTEROL (mg)	SODIUM (mg)	FIBER (g)
Whoppers®	18	190	30	2	1	7	7.0	0	100	0
York Peppermint Pattie®	1 (1.5 oz.)	170	34	2	0	3	2.0	0	10	0

CEREALS (Manufacturer's suggested serving)
Cooked, prepared w/ water

ITEM	AMOUNT	CALORIES	CARBOHYDRATE (g)	CARBOHYDRATE CHOICES	PROTEIN (g)	FAT (g)	SATURATED FAT (g)	CHOLESTEROL (mg)	SODIUM (mg)	FIBER (g)
Banana nut bread, instant	1 pkt.	150	32	2	3	2	0.0	0	210	3
Blueberry muffin, instant	1 pkt.	140	31	2	3	1	0.0	0	170	2
Coco Wheats®	1 cup	200	41	3	7	1	0.0	0	15	2
Cream of Rice®	1 cup	170	38	2½	3	0	0.0	0	0	0
Cream of Wheat®	1 cup	120	25	1½	3	0	0.0	0	0	1
Farina®	1 cup	120	22	1½	3	0	0.0	0	0	0
Grits, corn										
white, instant	1 pkt.	100	22	1½	2	0	0.0	0	300	1
white, regular	1 cup	140	32	2	3	1	0.0	0	0	2
yellow, regular	1 cup	120	29	2	3	0	0.0	0	0	2
Kashi Go®	½ cup	260	55	3	7	3	0.0	0	5	6
Malt-O-Meal®	1 cup	120	28	2	3	0	0.0	0	0	1
Maypo®	1 cup	190	36	2½	6	2	0.0	0	0	3
Oat bran	1 cup	150	25	1	7	3	0.5	0	0	6
Oatmeal										
raisins & spice, instant	1 pkt.	150	33	2	3	2	0.5	0	250	3
regular	1 cup	150	27	2	5	3	0.5	0	0	4
regular, instant	1 pkt.	100	19	1	4	2	0.0	0	80	3
Ralston®	1 cup	150	31	2	5	1	0.0	0	0	5
Wheatena®	1 cup	160	33	2	5	1	0.0	0	0	5
Ready to Eat										
100% Bran™	⅓ cup	80	23	1	4	1	0.0	0	120	8
All-Bran®										
extra fiber	½ cup	50	20	½	3	1	0.0	0	120	13
regular	½ cup	80	24	1	4	1	0.0	0	65	10
Alpha-Bits®, frosted	1 cup	130	27	2	3	2	0.0	0	210	1
Amaranth flakes	¾ cup	100	24	1½	3	0	0.0	0	90	4
Apple Jacks®	1 cup	120	30	2	1	0	0.0	0	150	1
Banana Nut Crunch®	1 cup	250	43	3	5	6	1.0	0	250	4
Basic 4®	1 cup	200	43	3	4	3	0.0	0	320	3
Blueberry Morning®	1¼ cups	210	43	3	4	3	0.0	0	270	2
Bran flakes	¾ cup	100	24	1	3	1	0.0	0	220	5
Cap'n Crunch®										
Crunch Berries®	¾ cup	100	22	1½	1	2	0.0	0	180	1
original	¾ cup	110	23	1½	1	2	0.5	0	200	1
Peanut Butter Crunch®	¾ cup	110	22	1½	2	3	0.5	0	200	1

CEREALS
Ready to Eat

ITEM	AMOUNT	CALORIES	CARBOHYDRATE (g)	CARBOHYDRATE CHOICES	PROTEIN (g)	FAT (g)	SATURATED FAT (g)	CHOLESTEROL (mg)	SODIUM (mg)	FIBER (g)
Cheerios®										
apple cinnamon	¾ cup	120	25	1½	2	2	0.0	0	160	1
frosted	1 cup	120	25	1½	2	1	0.0	0	210	1
honey nut	1 cup	120	24	1½	3	2	0.0	0	270	2
multi-grain plus	1 cup	110	24	1½	3	1	0.0	0	200	3
original	1 cup	110	22	1½	3	2	0.0	0	280	3
team	1 cup	120	25	1½	2	1	0.0	0	210	2
Chex®										
corn	1 cup	110	26	2	2	0	0.0	0	300	0
multi-bran	1 cup	200	49	3	4	2	0.0	0	360	7
rice	1¼ cups	120	27	2	2	0	0.0	0	290	0
wheat	1 cup	180	41	2½	5	2	0.0	0	420	5
Cinnamon Toast Crunch®	¾ cup	130	24	1½	1	4	0.5	0	210	1
Cocoa Krispies®	¾ cup	120	27	2	1	1	0.5	0	150	1
Cocoa Pebbles®	¾ cup	120	26	2	1	1	1.0	0	160	0
Cocoa Puffs®	1 cup	120	27	2	1	1	0.0	0	170	0
Cookie Crisp®	1 cup	120	26	2	1	1	0.0	0	180	0
Corn flakes	1 cup	100	24	1½	2	0	0.0	0	300	1
Corn Pops®	1 cup	120	28	2	1	0	0.0	0	120	0
Cracklin' Oat Bran®	¾ cup	190	35	2	4	7	1.5	0	170	6
Cranberry Almond Crunch®	1 cup	210	43	3	4	3	0.0	0	200	3
Crispix®	1 cup	110	25	1½	2	0	0.0	0	210	1
Fiber One®	½ cup	60	24	1	2	1	0.0	0	130	13
Flax Plus™	¾ cup	120	23	1	4	2	0.0	0	140	5
French Toast Crunch®	¾ cup	120	26	2	1	1	0.0	0	180	0
Froot Loops®	1 cup	120	28	2	2	1	1.0	0	150	1
Frosted Flakes™	¾ cup	120	28	2	1	0	0.0	0	150	1
Fruit & Fibre®										
dates, raisins & walnuts	1 cup	210	42	2½	4	3	0.0	0	280	5
peaches, raisins & almonds	1 cup	210	41	2½	4	3	0.0	0	280	5
Fruity Pebbles®	¾ cup	110	24	1½	0	1	0.0	0	160	0
Golden Crisp®	¾ cup	110	25	1½	1	0	0.0	0	40	0
Golden Grahams®	¾ cup	120	25	1½	1	1	0.0	0	270	1
Granola										
lowfat	½ cup	190	39	2½	4	3	0.5	0	120	3
regular	½ cup	251	38	2½	6	10	7.0	0	116	3
Grape-nuts®										
flakes	¾ cup	100	24	1½	3	1	0.0	0	140	3
original	½ cup	210	47	3	6	1	0.0	0	350	5
Great Grains®, crunchy pecan	⅔ cup	220	38	2½	5	6	1.0	0	210	4
Healthy Choice®										
multi-grain squares	1 cup	190	44	2½	5	1	0.0	0	5	5

CEREALS
Ready to Eat

ITEM	AMOUNT	CALORIES	CARBOHYDRATE (g)	CARBOHYDRATE CHOICES	PROTEIN (g)	FAT (g)	SATURATED FAT (g)	CHOLESTEROL (mg)	SODIUM (mg)	FIBER (g)
Healthy Choice® *(con't.)*										
raisin almond crunch	1 cup	210	45	2½	5	3	0.0	0	230	5
Honey Bunches of Oats®	¾ cup	120	25	1½	2	2	0.5	0	190	1
Honeycomb®	1⅓ cups	110	26	2	2	1	0.0	0	220	0
Just Right®, fruit & nut	1 cup	220	49	3	4	2	0.0	0	280	3
Kashi®										
Honey Puffed Kashi®	1 cup	120	25	1½	3	1	0.0	0	6	2
Kashi Good Friends®	¾ cup	90	24	1	3	1	0.0	0	70	8
Kashi Medley®	½ cup	100	20	1	4	1	0.0	0	50	2
Kashi Pillows®	¾ cup	200	45	3	3	1	0.0	0	50	2
Kix®										
Berry Berry Kix®	¾ cup	120	26	2	1	2	0.0	0	180	0
original	1⅓ cups	120	26	2	2	1	0.0	0	270	1
Life®	¾ cup	120	25	1½	3	2	0.0	0	160	2
Lucky Charms®	1 cup	120	25	1½	2	1	0.0	0	210	1
Mini-Wheats®										
apple cinnamon	¾ cup	180	44	2½	4	1	0.0	0	20	5
frosted, bite size	1 cup	200	48	3	6	1	0.0	0	5	6
frosted, regular	5 biscuits	180	41	2½	5	1	0.0	0	5	5
raisin	¾ cup	180	42	2½	5	1	0.0	0	5	5
strawberry	¾ cup	170	40	2	4	1	0.0	0	15	5
Mueslix®, w/ almonds	¾ cup	200	39	2	5	5	1.0	0	260	5
Nutri-grain®										
almond raisin	1¼ cups	180	38	2½	4	3	0.0	0	170	3
wheat	¾ cup	100	23	1½	3	1	0.0	0	210	4
Oat bran flakes	¾ cup	110	23	1½	4	1	0.0	0	270	4
Oatmeal Crisp®, raisin	1 cup	210	45	3	5	2	0.0	0	220	4
Oreo O's®	¾ cup	110	21	1½	1	3	0.5	0	150	1
Product 19®	1 cup	100	25	1½	2	0	0.0	0	210	1
Puffed rice	1 cup	50	12	1	1	0	0.0	0	0	0
Puffed wheat	1¼ cups	50	11	1	2	0	0.0	0	0	1
Raisin bran	1 cup	200	47	2½	6	2	0.0	0	370	8
Raisin nut bran	¾ cup	200	41	2½	4	4	0.5	0	250	5
Rice Krispies®	1¼ cups	120	29	2	2	0	0.0	0	320	0
Rice Krispies Treats®	¾ cup	120	26	2	1	2	0.0	0	190	0
Shredded Wheat™										
frosted, bite size	1 cup	190	44	2½	4	1	0.0	0	10	5
original	2 biscuits	160	38	2	5	1	0.0	0	0	5
Shredded Wheat 'N Bran®	1¼ cups	200	47	2½	7	1	0.0	0	0	8
Smacks®	¾ cup	100	24	1½	2	1	0.0	0	50	1
Smart Start®	1 cup	180	43	3	3	1	0.0	0	310	2
Special K®	1 cup	110	23	1½	6	0	0.0	0	220	1

CEREALS
Ready to Eat

ITEM	AMOUNT	CALORIES	CARBOHYDRATE (g)	CARBOHYDRATE CHOICES	PROTEIN (g)	FAT (g)	SATURATED FAT (g)	CHOLESTEROL (mg)	SODIUM (mg)	FIBER (g)
Sunrise Organic™	¾ cup	110	26	2	1	1	0.0	0	190	1
Toasted Oatmeal Squares™	1 cup	220	43	3	7	3	0.5	0	260	4
Total®										
corn flakes	1⅓ cups	110	26	2	2	0	0.0	0	200	0
raisin bran	1 cup	180	43	2½	4	1	0.0	0	240	5
whole grain	¾ cup	110	24	1½	3	1	0.5	0	200	3
Trix®	1 cup	120	26	2	1	2	0.0	0	200	1
Waffle Crisp®	1 cup	130	24	1½	2	3	0.0	0	120	0
Wheat germ	2 T.	50	6	½	4	1	0.0	0	0	2
Wheaties®										
Crispy Wheaties 'n Raisins®	1 cup	190	45	3	4	1	0.0	0	270	4
frosted	¾ cup	110	27	2	1	0	0.0	0	200	0
original	1 cup	110	24	1½	3	1	0.0	0	220	3

CHEESE

ITEM	AMOUNT	CALORIES	CARBOHYDRATE (g)	CARBOHYDRATE CHOICES	PROTEIN (g)	FAT (g)	SATURATED FAT (g)	CHOLESTEROL (mg)	SODIUM (mg)	FIBER (g)
American										
fat free	1 oz.	45	4	0	6	0	0.0	4	433	0
reduced fat	1 oz.	51	1	0	7	2	1.0	10	405	0
regular	1 oz.	106	0	0	6	9	6.0	27	405	0
American, singles										
fat free	1 slice	30	3	0	5	0	0.0	0	300	0
reduced fat	1 slice	50	2	0	4	3	2.0	10	300	0
regular	1 slice	60	2	0	3	5	3.0	15	240	0
Blue	1 oz.	101	1	0	6	8	6.0	30	395	0
Brick	1 oz.	111	0	0	6	9	6.0	30	192	0
Brie	1 oz.	95	0	0	6	8	5.0	28	178	0
Camembert	1 oz.	85	0	0	6	7	4.0	20	239	0
Caraway	1 oz.	107	1	0	7	8	5.0	26	196	0
Cheddar										
fat free	1 oz.	40	3	0	7	0	0.0	0	413	0
reduced fat	1 oz.	81	1	0	9	5	3.5	20	223	0
regular	1 oz.	111	1	0	7	9	6.0	30	182	0
regular, shredded	¼ cup	110	1	0	7	9	5.0	30	180	0
spread	2 T.	90	3	0	5	7	3.0	20	210	0
Cheez Whiz®										
light	2 T.	80	6	½	6	3	2.0	15	540	0
regular	2 T.	90	3	0	4	7	5.0	20	540	0
Colby	1 oz.	111	1	0	7	9	6.0	30	182	0
Cottage cheese										
1% fat	½ cup	82	3	0	14	1	1.0	5	459	0
2% fat	½ cup	101	4	0	15	2	1.0	9	459	0
fat free	½ cup	80	5	0	14	0	0.0	10	440	0

CHEESE

ITEM	AMOUNT	CALORIES	CARBOHYDRATE (g)	CARBOHYDRATE CHOICES	PROTEIN (g)	FAT (g)	SATURATED FAT (g)	CHOLESTEROL (mg)	SODIUM (mg)	FIBER (g)
Cream cheese										
fat free	2 T.	30	2	0	5	0	0.0	3	160	0
light	2 T.	70	2	0	3	5	3.5	15	150	0
regular	2 T.	101	1	0	2	10	6.5	32	86	0
Cream cheese, flavored										
garden vegetable, regular	2 T.	110	1	0	1	11	7.0	30	170	0
roasted garlic, light	2 T.	70	2	0	3	5	3.5	15	180	0
strawberry, fat free	2 T.	45	6	½	4	0	0.0	0	190	0
Edam	1 oz.	101	0	0	7	8	5.0	25	274	0
Feta	1 oz.	81	1	0	5	6	4.5	25	314	0
Fondue	¼ cup	123	2	0	8	7	5.0	24	71	0
Fontina	1 oz.	98	0	0	6	8	4.0	25	171	0
Goat, soft	1 oz.	76	0	0	5	6	4.0	13	104	0
Gorgonzola	1 oz.	98	1	0	6	8	5.0	30	284	0
Gouda	1 oz.	111	1	0	7	9	6.0	25	162	0
Gruyere	1 oz.	117	0	0	8	9	5.5	31	95	0
Havarti	1 oz.	105	1	0	7	8	5.5	27	159	0
Healthy Choice®, singles	1 slice	40	2	0	5	1	0.5	0	200	0
Jarlsberg	1 oz.	107	1	0	8	8	5.0	26	74	0
Limburger	1 oz.	91	0	0	6	8	5.0	25	243	0
Mascarpone	1 oz.	126	1	0	2	13	7.0	36	16	0
Monterey Jack	1 oz.	111	0	0	6	9	6.0	30	192	0
Mozzarella										
part-skim	1 oz.	79	1	0	8	5	3.0	15	150	0
whole milk	1 oz.	90	0	0	6	7	4.5	20	106	0
Muenster	1 oz.	111	0	0	6	9	6.0	30	192	0
Neufchatel	1 oz.	74	1	0	3	7	4.0	22	113	0
Parmesan										
grated	1 T.	29	0	0	3	2	1.0	5	116	0
grated, fat free	1 T.	23	5	0	0	0	0.0	0	113	0
hard, shredded	1 T.	21	0	0	2	1	1.0	4	85	0
Pepper Jack	1 oz.	111	1	0	7	9	6.0	30	192	0
Port wine, cold pack										
light	2 T.	70	5	0	5	4	2.0	15	190	0
regular	2 T.	90	3	0	5	7	3.0	20	210	0
Provolone	1 oz.	100	1	0	7	8	5.0	20	248	0
Ricotta										
fat free	½ cup	120	10	½	20	0	0.0	0	120	0
lowfat	½ cup	140	6	½	12	6	3.0	32	90	0
part-skim	½ cup	170	6	½	14	10	6.0	38	154	0
whole milk	½ cup	214	4	0	14	16	10.0	62	103	0
Romano	1 oz.	100	1	0	8	8	4.5	20	390	0

CHEESE

ITEM	AMOUNT	CALORIES	CARBOHYDRATE (g)	CARBOHYDRATE CHOICES	PROTEIN (g)	FAT (g)	SATURATED FAT (g)	CHOLESTEROL (mg)	SODIUM (mg)	FIBER (g)
Roquefort	1 oz.	105	1	0	6	9	5.5	26	513	0
Soy cheese	1 oz.	40	2	0	6	3	0.0	0	80	0
String cheese	1 oz.	72	1	0	7	5	3.0	16	132	0
Swiss										
natural	1 oz.	100	1	0	8	8	5.0	25	60	0
processed	1 oz.	111	0	0	8	9	6.0	30	320	0
Velveeta®										
light	1 oz.	60	3	0	5	3	2.0	10	440	0
regular	1 oz.	90	3	0	5	6	4.0	25	420	0
Yogurt cheese	1 oz.	22	3	0	2	0	0.0	1	22	0

COMBINATION FOODS, FROZEN ENTRÉES & MEALS

Homemade unless indicated

ITEM	AMOUNT	CALORIES	CARBOHYDRATE (g)	CARBOHYDRATE CHOICES	PROTEIN (g)	FAT (g)	SATURATED FAT (g)	CHOLESTEROL (mg)	SODIUM (mg)	FIBER (g)
Bagel Bites®, frzn.										
cheese	4	190	25	1½	9	6	3.5	15	530	1
pepperoni	4	200	26	2	9	7	3.5	15	610	1
Baked beans, can										
w/ franks	½ cup	183	20	1	9	9	3.0	8	553	4
w/ pork	½ cup	134	25	1	7	2	1.0	9	522	7
Beans & rice, box	½ cup	120	24	1	5	0	0.0	0	590	5
Beef goulash, w/ noodles	1 cup	341	23	1½	30	14	3.5	88	457	2
Beef Oriental	1 cup	104	12	1	10	2	0.5	12	969	4
Beef stroganoff, w/ noodles	1 cup	342	21	1½	20	20	7.5	73	454	2
Beefaroni®, can	1 cup	260	37	2	10	7	3.0	25	870	5
Burritos, frzn.										
bean	1 (5 oz.)	290	44	3	12	9	4.5	15	840	3
beef	1 (6 oz.)	405	45	3	21	16	8.0	49	1153	1
chicken	1 (6 oz.)	345	41	3	17	13	5.0	57	854	1
Casseroles										
chicken & noodles	1 cup	326	29	2	23	13	4.0	84	732	2
green bean	1 cup	300	22	1½	6	20	6.0	10	1240	4
hamburger & macaroni	1 cup	216	31	2	14	4	4.0	28	847	2
seafood Newburg	1 cup	612	11	1	30	50	30.0	424	892	0
tuna noodle	1 cup	237	25	1½	17	7	2.0	41	772	1
Chicken à la king	1 cup	468	12	1	27	34	13.0	186	760	1
Chicken cacciatore	6 oz.	319	9	½	29	18	4.0	89	412	2
Chicken cordon bleu	6 oz.	358	6	½	34	21	11.0	142	458	0
Chicken divan	6 oz.	228	6	½	29	10	4.0	96	289	2
Chicken Helper®, box										
chicken & herb	1 cup	260	24	1½	3	7	1.5	60	490	0
creamy roasted garlic	1 cup	290	27	2	5	8	2.5	65	650	1

COMBINATION FOODS, FROZEN ENTRÉES & MEALS

ITEM	AMOUNT	CALORIES	CARBOHYDRATE (g)	CARBOHYDRATE CHOICES	PROTEIN (g)	FAT (g)	SATURATED FAT (g)	CHOLESTEROL (mg)	SODIUM (mg)	FIBER (g)
Chicken Helper®, box *(con't.)*										
fettucini Alfredo	1 cup	300	28	2	27	9	3.5	65	870	1
Chicken nuggets, frzn.	4	210	9	½	11	15	3.5	35	300	1
Chicken parmigiana	6 oz.	296	14	1	27	15	5.0	129	717	1
Chicken tetrazzini	1 cup	372	28	2	19	20	7.0	50	813	2
Chili, w/ beans, can										
beef	1 cup	270	33	2	18	7	3.0	35	1240	7
turkey	1 cup	210	30	1½	17	3	1.0	35	1180	5
vegetarian	1 cup	200	38	2	12	1	0.0	0	780	7
Chimichangas, frzn.										
beef	1 (4.5 oz.)	370	37	2½	9	20	5.0	10	470	3
chicken	1 (4.5 oz.)	350	39	2½	11	16	4.0	20	540	2
Chipped beef, creamed	1 cup	350	18	1	18	23	8.0	44	1467	0
Chop suey, can										
beef	1 cup	275	12	1	22	16	4.0	54	774	2
chicken	1 cup	194	10	½	20	8	2.0	49	967	2
pork	1 cup	287	12	1	22	17	4.5	56	771	2
Chow mein, can										
beef	1 cup	90	9	½	10	2	0.5	15	830	2
chicken	1 cup	95	18	1	7	1	0.0	8	725	2
Corn dogs, frzn.	1 (2.8 oz.)	220	25	1½	6	11	3.0	45	520	1
Create a Meal!®, frzn.										
BBQ chicken	1⅓ cups	350	37	2½	29	9	1.5	65	1340	4
cheesy pasta & vegetables	1¼ cups	420	29	2	29	21	10.0	95	1350	2
chicken & stuffing	1⅓ cups	370	36	2½	31	11	1.5	60	1540	2
Szechuan stir-fry	1¼ cups	310	20	1	26	14	3.0	60	1390	4
Egg rolls, frzn.										
pork	1 (2 oz.)	170	23	1½	6	6	1.5	5	390	3
shrimp	1 (2 oz.)	150	24	1½	6	4	0.5	10	420	3
Eggplant parmigiana	1 cup	320	17	1	15	22	10.0	57	684	3
Enchiladas										
beef	1 (6 oz.)	286	27	2	11	16	8.0	36	1169	2
chicken	1 (6 oz.)	272	22	1½	19	12	5.0	51	436	3
Fajitas										
beef	1 (6 in.)	156	18	1	7	7	2.0	10	325	2
chicken	1 (6 in.)	155	19	1	9	5	1.0	16	168	2
Frozen breakfasts										
burrito, ham & cheese	1 (3.5 oz.)	212	28	2	10	7	2.0	192	405	1
egg & cheese sandwich	1 (4.1 oz.)	290	25	1½	14	15	6.0	95	750	2
eggs, w/ bacon	1 (5.3 oz.)	290	17	1	11	19	9.0	240	700	1
eggs, w/ home fries	1 (4.4 oz.)	200	15	1	7	12	8.0	190	390	2
eggs, w/ sausage	1 (6.2 oz.)	360	21	1½	12	26	10.0	280	800	3

COMBINATION FOODS, FROZEN ENTRÉES & MEALS

ITEM	AMOUNT	CALORIES	CARBOHYDRATE (g)	CARBOHYDRATE CHOICES	PROTEIN (g)	FAT (g)	SATURATED FAT (g)	CHOLESTEROL (mg)	SODIUM (mg)	FIBER (g)
Frozen breakfasts *(con't.)*										
French toast, w/ sausage	1 (5.5 oz.)	410	33	2	13	26	9.0	110	580	3
pancakes, w/ bacon	1 (4.5 oz.)	400	42	3	12	20	7.0	100	1030	1
pancakes, w/ sausage	1 (6 oz.)	490	52	3½	14	25	11.0	90	950	3
Frozen dinners										
beef tips, w/ noodles	1 (10 oz.)	290	34	2	16	11	5.0	50	530	5
chicken, fried	1 (11 oz.)	430	49	3	23	16	4.5	40	1010	5
chicken & dumplings	1 (10 oz.)	260	35	2	13	8	2.5	35	780	3
chicken cordon bleu	1 (13 oz.)	590	58	3½	33	25	8.0	55	1920	7
chicken fried steak	1 (15 oz.)	650	69	4	23	31	10.0	50	2260	7
chicken Marsala	1 (14 oz.)	450	42	2½	33	17	7.0	70	1260	6
chicken parmigiana	1 (11 oz.)	370	40	2½	13	17	5.0	25	1010	4
chopped sirloin	1 (11 oz.)	380	37	2	19	14	6.0	40	730	5
fish 'n chips	1 (10 oz.)	490	59	3½	19	20	4.0	45	1030	5
meatloaf	1 (11 oz.)	493	58	3½	19	22	7.0	79	1724	5
pork rib, boneless	1 (11 oz.)	470	58	3½	16	19	7.0	30	900	5
pot roast	1 (11 oz.)	250	39	2	12	5	1.5	20	850	5
Salisbury steak, w/ gravy	1 (14 oz.)	550	51	3	30	25	11.0	85	1680	6
Swedish meatballs	1 (9 oz.)	440	36	2½	23	23	8.0	85	840	3
Swiss steak	1 (11 oz.)	413	42	2½	22	17	6.0	64	765	5
turkey	1 (9 oz.)	270	31	2	15	10	3.0	45	1100	3
veal parmigiana	1 (11 oz.)	390	40	2	19	18	8.0	85	1060	5
Frozen dinners, Healthy Choice®										
pepper steak Oriental	1 (10 oz.)	260	34	2	19	5	2.5	35	520	2
roasted chicken	1 (11 oz.)	230	25	1	20	5	2.5	45	480	6
stuffed pasta shells	1 (10 oz.)	370	60	3½	18	6	3.0	20	570	5
Frozen entrées										
chicken & dumplings	1 (10 oz.)	280	33	2	19	8	3.5	55	1000	0
fettucini primavera	1 (10 oz.)	430	49	3	13	20	12.0	50	1100	5
manicotti, w/ red sauce	1 (9 oz.)	380	38	2½	18	17	9.0	45	880	4
meatloaf	1 (10 oz.)	330	26	2	20	16	6.0	70	850	3
turkey	1 (10 oz.)	320	31	2	19	13	3.5	50	950	3
Frozen entrées, Lean Cuisine®										
Alfredo pasta primavera	1 (10 oz.)	290	46	3	11	7	3.0	10	570	3
chicken teriyaki	1 (10 oz.)	290	48	3	17	4	0.5	25	590	4
oven roasted beef	1 (9.3 oz.)	260	28	2	18	8	3.0	50	590	4
penne pasta	1 (10 oz.)	270	52	3	8	4	1.0	0	350	5
Hamburger Helper®, box										
beef pasta	1 cup	270	26	2	20	10	4.0	50	910	1
cheeseburger macaroni	1 cup	360	31	2	23	16	6.0	65	1000	1
Italian rigatoni	1 cup	180	29	2	19	10	4.0	50	870	1

COMBINATION FOODS, FROZEN ENTRÉES & MEALS

ITEM	AMOUNT	CALORIES	CARBOHYDRATE (g)	CARBOHYDRATE CHOICES	PROTEIN (g)	FAT (g)	SATURATED FAT (g)	CHOLESTEROL (mg)	SODIUM (mg)	FIBER (g)
Hot Pockets®, frzn.										
chicken, cheddar & broccoli	1 (4.5 oz.)	300	40	2½	13	10	5.0	40	510	2
ham & cheddar	1 (4.5 oz.)	320	39	2½	14	12	6.0	45	790	2
Philly steak & cheese	1 (4.5 oz.)	350	37	2½	15	16	8.0	50	790	2
Lasagna										
w/ meat	1 cup	354	36	2½	21	14	7.0	52	690	3
w/ vegetables	1 cup	310	40	2½	16	10	5.5	32	743	3
Lean Pockets®, frzn.	1 (4.5 oz.)	280	41	3	11	7	3.0	35	570	2
Lo mein, pork	1 cup	323	36	2½	19	12	2.0	34	313	3
Macaroni & cheese										
box	1 cup	390	48	3	11	17	4.0	10	730	1
frozen	1 cup	320	31	2	13	16	7.0	30	990	3
Manicotti, w/ red sauce	2 (5 in.)	340	32	1½	18	16	7.0	50	810	7
Meatballs	1 (1 oz.)	60	2	0	5	4	1.5	23	106	0
Meatloaf	3 oz.	181	5	0	14	11	4.0	71	322	0
Moussaka	1 cup	237	13	1	16	13	4.5	97	432	4
Pepper steak	1 cup	331	5	0	29	21	4.0	73	650	1
Pizzas, French bread, frzn.										
cheese	1 (5.2 oz.)	370	43	3	14	16	6.0	15	880	3
cheese, Healthy Choice®	1 (6 oz.)	340	51	3	22	5	1.5	15	480	5
pepperoni	1 (5.6 oz.)	390	48	3	14	16	6.0	25	840	4
Pizzas, frzn.										
pepperoni	1 slice	340	29	2	15	18	8.0	35	750	2
three cheese	1 slice	380	25	1½	20	22	12.0	45	730	2
vegetable	1 slice	240	31	2	25	7	2.5	10	500	3
Pizza Rolls®, frzn.										
cheese	6	210	25	1½	9	8	2.5	10	420	1
pepperoni	6	240	24	1½	8	12	3.0	15	550	1
Pot pies, frzn.										
beef	1 (8 oz.)	449	42	3	17	27	7.0	42	856	3
beef/chicken, Hungry-Man®	1 (14 oz.)	690	66	4	20	38	14.0	45	1430	6
chicken	1 (7 oz.)	410	45	3	9	22	8.0	30	810	3
Ravioli, w/ red sauce										
cheese	1 cup	310	41	3	12	11	4.0	20	1150	2
meat	1 cup	352	33	2	19	16	5.5	153	1123	2
Salmon loaf	3 oz.	170	7	½	13	9	2.5	99	641	0
Salmon patties	1 (4 oz.)	261	14	1	16	16	4.0	56	657	1
Sandwiches, w/ bread/bun										
BBQ beef	1 (6 oz.)	387	41	3	28	11	4.0	63	641	3
BLT, w/ mayo.	1 (4.5 oz.)	336	33	2	11	18	4.0	22	630	2
bologna & cheese	1 (4 oz.)	363	26	2	13	22	10.0	42	1009	1
bratwurst	1 (4.5 oz.)	370	22	1½	15	24	8.0	51	697	1

COMBINATION FOODS, FROZEN ENTRÉES & MEALS

ITEM	AMOUNT	CALORIES	CARBOHYDRATE (g)	CARBOHYDRATE CHOICES	PROTEIN (g)	FAT (g)	SATURATED FAT (g)	CHOLESTEROL (mg)	SODIUM (mg)	FIBER (g)
Sandwiches, w/ bread/bun *(con't.)*										
cheeseburger	1 (5 oz.)	380	28	2	23	19	9.0	65	770	1
chicken, breaded & fried	1 (6 oz.)	383	33	2	21	18	3.5	49	677	2
chicken, broiled	1 (6 oz.)	287	28	2	22	9	2.0	46	961	3
chicken salad, w/ mayo.	1 (4 oz.)	379	34	2	11	22	3.5	32	475	2
club, w/ mayo.	1 (6 oz.)	370	35	2	24	16	3.0	55	764	2
corned beef & Swiss	1 (6 oz.)	458	24	1½	30	28	10.0	89	1518	2
egg salad, w/ mayo.	1 (4 oz.)	369	32	2	10	22	4.0	142	511	1
grilled cheese	1 (4 oz.)	380	30	2	17	21	11.5	50	1049	1
ham & cheese, w/ mustard	1 (6 oz.)	444	36	2½	24	22	8.5	63	1705	2
ham salad, w/ mayo.	1 (4 oz.)	316	33	2	9	16	4.0	25	776	1
hamburger	1 (5 oz.)	298	30	2	17	12	5.0	46	647	2
hot dog	1 (3.5 oz.)	241	19	1	9	14	5.0	25	732	1
peanut butter & jelly	1 (4 oz.)	368	50	3	13	15	3.0	0	373	6
roast beef, w/ mayo.	1 (6 oz.)	437	37	2½	32	18	3.5	49	1728	1
Rueben, w/ dressing	1 (6 oz.)	496	31	2	23	31	10.5	89	1309	4
salami & cheese, w/ mustard	1 (4 oz.)	356	24	1½	16	21	10.0	51	974	1
sloppy Joe, beef	1 (4 oz.)	392	39	2½	20	17	6.0	54	1056	3
tuna salad, w/ mayo.	1 (4 oz.)	308	34	2	13	13	2.0	13	524	2
turkey, w/ mustard	1 (6 oz.)	337	36	2½	27	8	1.5	44	1714	2
Scalloped potatoes & ham	1 cup	234	26	2	12	10	6.0	38	1077	2
Shepherd's pie	1 cup	287	31	2	18	10	3.0	41	702	3
Skillet Sensations™, frzn.										
chicken Alfredo	1½ cups	490	63	3½	23	16	6.0	30	1240	9
chicken & grilled vegetables	1½ cups	440	62	4	27	9	4.0	30	1330	6
homestyle beef	1½ cups	360	34	2	30	11	5.0	70	1090	4
Skillet Sensations™, Lean Cuisine®, frzn.										
chicken Oriental	1½ cups	280	46	2½	17	3	0.5	15	750	6
roast beef & potatoes	1½ cups	290	38	2	18	7	3.0	35	760	9
roasted turkey	1½ cups	220	37	2	14	2	0.5	25	790	6
Spaghetti, w/ meatballs	1 cup	332	39	2	19	12	3.0	74	1009	8
SpaghettiO's®, can										
w/ meatballs	1 cup	260	31	2	11	11	5.0	20	1150	5
w/ tomato sauce	1 cup	190	36	2½	5	2	0.5	5	990	2
Stew										
beef, can	1 cup	194	17	1	14	8	2.5	34	1007	2
beef, hmde.	1 cup	218	15	1	16	11	5.0	64	292	2
chicken, can	1 cup	220	16	1	12	11	3.0	40	980	2
Stuffed cabbage rolls	1 (6 oz.)	134	17	1	6	5	1.0	9	414	3
Stuffed green peppers	1 (6 oz.)	229	20	1	11	11	5.0	34	201	2
Stuffed shells, w/ red sauce	2 (3 oz.)	390	38	2½	17	21	11.0	100	805	2
Sweet & sour pork	1 cup	231	25	1½	15	8	2.0	38	1120	1

COMBINATION FOODS, FROZEN ENTRÉES & MEALS

ITEM	AMOUNT	CALORIES	CARBOHYDRATE (g)	CARBOHYDRATE CHOICES	PROTEIN (g)	FAT (g)	SATURATED FAT (g)	CHOLESTEROL (mg)	SODIUM (mg)	FIBER (g)
Tacos, beef/chicken	1 (3 oz.)	190	11	1	11	12	5.0	35	297	1
Tamales	1 (2.4 oz.)	110	10	½	2	6	2.5	10	197	2
Tortellini, w/ red sauce										
cheese	1 cup	470	65	4	22	15	7.0	75	945	4
meat	1 cup	450	67	4½	22	11	3.0	45	715	4
Tuna Helper®, box										
Alfredo	1 cup	310	32	2	14	14	3.5	15	950	1
au gratin	1 cup	310	36	2½	14	12	3.0	20	930	1
tuna pot pie	1 cup	440	40	2½	18	24	7.0	110	1080	1
Veal Marsala	6 oz.	467	11	1	22	34	14.5	117	365	0
Veal parmigiana	6 oz.	350	21	1½	27	17	6.0	86	1627	1
Veal scallopini	6 oz.	456	2	0	31	34	10.0	110	675	0
Welsh rarebit, frzn.	1 cup	439	18	1	18	33	14.5	73	1024	0
Yorkshire pudding	2 oz.	118	14	1	4	6	2.5	43	335	1
Ziti, w/ meat sauce	1 cup	354	36	2½	21	14	7.0	52	690	3

CONDIMENTS, SAUCES, & BAKING INGREDIENTS

Condiments & Sauces

ITEM	AMOUNT	CALORIES	CARBOHYDRATE (g)	CARBOHYDRATE CHOICES	PROTEIN (g)	FAT (g)	SATURATED FAT (g)	CHOLESTEROL (mg)	SODIUM (mg)	FIBER (g)
Alfredo sauce	¼ cup	230	2	0	4	22	10.0	45	550	0
BBQ sauce	1 T.	20	5	0	0	0	0.0	0	230	0
Béarnaise sauce	2 T.	80	0	0	1	8	5.0	59	111	0
Béchamel sauce	2 T.	35	2	0	0	3	2.0	8	281	0
Catsup/ketchup	1 T.	15	4	0	0	0	0.0	0	190	0
Cheese sauce	2 T.	55	2	0	3	4	2.0	9	129	0
Chili sauce	2 T.	35	8	½	1	0	0.0	0	456	0
Chutney	2 T.	52	13	1	0	0	0.0	0	76	1
Clam sauce										
red	½ cup	60	8	½	4	1	0.0	10	350	1
white	½ cup	130	1	0	10	9	1.5	15	310	0
Cocktail sauce	2 T.	30	7	½	1	0	0.0	0	400	0
Cranberry sauce	2 T.	52	13	1	0	0	0.0	0	10	0
Cranberry-orange relish	2 T.	61	16	1	0	0	0.0	0	11	0
Duck sauce	2 T.	70	18	1	0	0	0.0	0	180	0
Enchilada sauce										
green	2 T.	22	2	0	0	2	1.0	5	46	0
red	2 T.	41	2	0	0	4	2.0	11	42	0
Fish sauce	1 T.	6	1	0	1	0	0.0	0	1390	0
Hoisin sauce	1 T.	35	7	½	1	1	0.0	0	258	0
Hollandaise sauce	2 T.	85	0	0	1	9	5.0	90	78	0
Horseradish	1 T.	6	1	0	0	0	0.0	0	14	0
Horseradish sauce	1 T.	29	1	0	0	3	2.0	6	41	0

CONDIMENTS, SAUCES & BAKING INGREDIENTS
Condiments & Sauces

ITEM	AMOUNT	CALORIES	CARBOHYDRATE (g)	CARBOHYDRATE CHOICES	PROTEIN (g)	FAT (g)	SATURATED FAT (g)	CHOLESTEROL (mg)	SODIUM (mg)	FIBER (g)
Lobster sauce	1 T.	24	1	0	1	2	0.0	10	121	0
Manwich® sauce	¼ cup	30	6	½	0	0	0.0	0	360	0
Mole poblana sauce	2 T.	50	4	0	1	3	1.0	0	41	1
Mornay sauce	2 T.	92	3	0	3	8	4.0	40	201	0
Mustard										
brown/yellow	1 tsp.	5	0	0	0	0	0.0	0	65	0
Dijon	1 tsp.	5	0	0	0	0	0.0	0	120	0
honey-mustard	1 tsp.	17	2	0	0	1	0.0	0	30	0
Olives										
black	5	25	1	0	0	2	0.0	0	192	1
green	5	23	0	0	0	2	0.0	0	468	0
Oyster sauce	1 T.	30	6	½	0	0	0.0	0	900	0
Pasta sauce, red										
four cheese, Classico®	½ cup	80	8	½	2	4	1.0	0	500	1
light, Ragú®	½ cup	60	9	½	3	2	0.0	0	390	3
marinara, hmde.	½ cup	94	13	1	2	5	1.0	0	657	3
meat flavored, Ragú®	½ cup	80	8	½	2	4	0.5	0	880	2
Sockarooni™, Newman's Own®	½ cup	60	9	½	2	2	0.0	0	590	3
tomato & basil, Barilla®	½ cup	70	12	1	2	2	0.5	0	640	3
traditional, Healthy Choice®	½ cup	50	11	1	3	0	0.0	0	390	2
traditional, Prego®	½ cup	140	23	1½	2	5	1.5	0	610	2
w/ meat, hmde.	½ cup	144	11	1	8	8	2.0	23	565	2
Peanut sauce	2 T.	93	4	0	4	8	1.5	0	74	1
Pesto sauce	2 T.	155	2	0	5	14	4.0	9	211	0
Pickles										
dill/sour	1 medium	7	1	0	1	0	0.0	0	928	1
sweet	1 medium	41	11	1	0	0	0.0	0	329	1
Pico de gallo	2 T.	5	2	0	0	0	0.0	0	260	1
Pizza sauce	¼ cup	24	4	0	1	1	0.0	0	288	1
Plum sauce	2 T.	46	11	1	0	0	0.0	0	133	0
Relish, sweet pickle	1 T.	21	5	0	0	0	0.0	0	109	0
Salsa	2 T.	11	2	0	0	0	0.0	0	251	0
Salt	1 tsp.	0	0	0	0	0	0.0	0	2325	0
Sauerkraut	2 T.	6	1	0	0	0	0.0	0	195	1
Soy sauce										
lite	1 T.	15	2	0	1	0	0.0	0	505	0
regular	1 T.	11	1	0	1	0	0.0	0	1315	0
Spices, salt free	¼ tsp.	0	0	0	0	0	0.0	0	0	0
Steak sauce										
A.1.®	1 T.	15	3	0	0	0	0.0	0	280	0
Heinz 57®	1 T.	15	4	0	0	0	0.0	0	220	0
Stir-fry sauce	1 T.	14	3	0	1	0	0.0	0	369	0

CONDIMENTS, SAUCES & BAKING INGREDIENTS

Condiments & Sauces

ITEM	AMOUNT	CALORIES	CARBOHYDRATE (g)	CARBOHYDRATE CHOICES	PROTEIN (g)	FAT (g)	SATURATED FAT (g)	CHOLESTEROL (mg)	SODIUM (mg)	FIBER (g)
Stroganoff sauce	2 T.	28	4	0	1	1	1.0	4	191	0
Sweet & sour sauce	1 T.	25	7	½	0	0	0.0	0	190	0
Szechuan sauce	1 T.	12	2	0	0	0	0.0	0	127	0
Tabasco® sauce	1 tsp.	0	0	0	0	0	0.0	0	30	0
Taco sauce	1 T.	10	2	0	0	0	0.0	0	125	0
Tamari sauce	1 T.	10	1	0	2	0	0.0	0	930	0
Tartar sauce	1 T.	74	1	0	0	8	1.5	7	99	0
Teriyaki sauce	1 T.	15	3	0	1	0	0.0	0	690	0
Tomato sauce	½ cup	37	9	½	2	0	0.0	0	741	2
Vinegar										
balsamic	1 T.	10	2	0	0	0	0.0	0	4	0
cider/white	1 T.	2	1	0	0	0	0.0	0	0	0
raspberry/red wine	1 T.	0	0	0	0	0	0.0	0	0	0
White cream sauce	2 T.	30	2	0	1	2	1.0	3	140	0
Worcestershire sauce	1 tsp.	4	1	0	0	0	0.0	0	56	0
Baking Ingredients										
Baking powder	¼ tsp.	0	0	0	0	0	0.0	0	95	0
Baking soda	¼ tsp.	0	0	0	0	0	0.0	0	315	0
Bisquick®, mix, dry										
reduced fat	½ cup	227	42	3	5	4	1.0	0	697	1
regular	½ cup	245	37	2½	4	9	2.5	0	756	1
Bread crumbs										
plain	¼ cup	100	19	1	4	2	0.0	0	210	1
seasoned	¼ cup	110	21	1½	4	1	0.0	1	795	1
Butterscotch chips	1 T.	80	9	½	0	4	3.5	0	15	0
Carob chips, unsweetened	1 T.	35	4	0	1	2	1.5	0	25	1
Chocolate, baking										
semi-sweet	1 oz.	142	18	1	2	8	5.0	0	0	4
unsweetened	1 oz.	148	8	½	3	16	9.0	0	4	4
Chocolate chips										
milk chocolate	1 T.	70	9	½	0	4	2.5	0	0	0
semi-sweet	1 T.	70	9	½	0	4	2.0	0	0	0
Cocoa powder	1 T.	15	3	0	1	1	0.0	0	0	2
Corn flake crumbs	¼ cup	80	18	1	2	0	0.0	0	240	0
Corn starch	1 T.	30	7	½	0	0	0.0	0	1	0
Corn syrup, dark/light	1 T.	58	16	1	0	0	0.0	0	32	0
Cornmeal	2 T.	55	12	1	1	1	0.0	0	5	1
Flour										
all purpose/white	1 cup	455	95	6	13	1	0.0	0	3	3
bread	1 cup	433	87	6	16	2	0.5	0	1	3
buckwheat	1 cup	400	84	5	16	4	0.0	0	0	12
cake	1 cup	496	107	7	11	1	0.0	0	3	2

CONDIMENTS, SAUCES & BAKING INGREDIENTS
Baking Ingredients

ITEM	AMOUNT	CALORIES	CARBOHYDRATE (g)	CARBOHYDRATE CHOICES	PROTEIN (g)	FAT (g)	SATURATED FAT (g)	CHOLESTEROL (mg)	SODIUM (mg)	FIBER (g)
Flour *(con't.)*										
carob	1 cup	229	92	4½	5	1	0.0	0	36	24
corn	1 cup	422	90	5	8	5	0.5	0	6	16
potato	1 cup	639	149	9	12	1	0.0	0	98	11
rice, white	1 cup	578	127	8½	9	2	0.5	0	0	4
rye, medium	1 cup	401	86	5	10	2	0.5	0	0	10
soy	1 cup	369	27	1	32	18	2.5	0	11	8
soy, fat free	1 cup	329	38	2	47	1	0.0	0	20	8
white, self-rising	1 cup	443	93	6	12	1	0.0	0	1588	3
whole wheat	1 cup	407	87	5	16	2	0.5	0	6	15
Graham cracker crumbs	¼ cup	127	23	1½	2	3	0.5	0	182	1
Honey	1 T.	64	17	1	0	0	0.0	0	0	0
Lighter Bake™	1 T.	35	9	½	0	0	0.0	0	0	0
Matzo meal, unsalted	2 T.	65	14	1	2	0	0.0	0	0	0
Molasses	1 T.	55	14	1	0	0	0.0	0	8	0
Phyllo dough	8 sheets	180	35	2	5	1	0.0	0	300	1
Pie crusts										
graham	⅛ pie	130	17	1	1	6	1.5	0	170	0
pastry, double	⅛ pie	211	19	1	3	14	3.5	0	217	1
pastry, single	⅛ pie	119	11	1	1	8	2.0	0	122	0
Pie fillings										
apple	½ cup	129	33	2	0	0	0.0	0	56	1
cherry	½ cup	152	39	2½	1	0	0.0	0	12	1
lemon	½ cup	140	29	2	1	2	0.5	0	75	0
Shake 'n Bake®, box	¼ pkt.	80	13	1	2	2	0.0	0	350	0
Sugar										
brown/raw/white	1 cup	774	200	13	0	0	0.0	0	2	0
powdered	1 cup	467	119	8	0	0	0.0	0	1	0
Yeast	1 pkt.	21	3	0	3	0	0.0	0	4	1

CRACKERS, DIPS & SNACK FOODS
Crackers

ITEM	AMOUNT	CALORIES	CARBOHYDRATE (g)	CARBOHYDRATE CHOICES	PROTEIN (g)	FAT (g)	SATURATED FAT (g)	CHOLESTEROL (mg)	SODIUM (mg)	FIBER (g)
Air Crisps®										
cheese	32	130	21	1½	3	4	1.0	0	300	0
potato	24	120	21	1½	2	4	0.5	0	210	1
Ritz®	24	140	22	1½	2	5	1.0	0	240	0
Ak-mak®	5	116	19	1	5	2	0.5	0	214	4
Animal										
iced	6	150	24	1½	2	5	1.0	0	110	0
plain	6	84	14	1	1	2	0.5	0	90	0
Cheese, w/ peanut butter	4	140	16	1	3	8	1.5	0	210	0

CRACKERS, DIPS & SNACK FOODS
Crackers

ITEM	AMOUNT	CALORIES	CARBOHYDRATE (g)	CARBOHYDRATE CHOICES	PROTEIN (g)	FAT (g)	SATURATED FAT (g)	CHOLESTEROL (mg)	SODIUM (mg)	FIBER (g)
Cheez-It®										
reduced fat	29	140	20	1	4	5	1.0	0	240	0
regular	27	160	16	1	4	8	2.0	0	240	0
Chicken In A Biskit®	12	160	17	1	2	9	1.5	0	270	0
Club®										
reduced fat	5	70	12	1	1	2	0.0	0	200	0
regular	4	70	9	½	1	3	1.0	0	160	0
Gold Fish®	55	140	19	1	3	6	2.0	0	230	0
Graham										
reduced fat	2 sheets	110	23	1½	2	2	0.0	0	200	0
regular	2 sheets	120	22	1½	2	3	0.0	0	180	1
sugar free, Estee®	2 sheets	90	17	1	3	2	0.0	0	115	2
Harvest Crisps®	13	130	23	1½	3	4	0.5	0	270	1
Matzoh	1 sheet	110	24	1½	3	0	0.0	0	60	1
Melba snacks	5	60	12	1	2	1	0.0	0	135	2
Oyster	23	60	11	1	1	2	0.0	0	230	1
Ritz®										
low sodium	5	80	10	½	1	4	0.5	0	35	0
reduced fat	5	70	11	1	1	2	0.0	0	140	0
regular	5	80	10	½	1	4	0.5	0	135	0
Ritz Bits® sandwiches	14	170	17	1	3	10	2.5	5	300	0
Saltines										
fat free	5	60	12	1	2	0	0.0	0	180	0
low sodium	5	65	11	1	1	2	0.0	0	95	0
regular	5	60	10	½	1	2	0.0	0	180	0
Seasoned Ry Krisp®	2	60	10	½	1	2	0.0	0	90	3
SnackWell's®										
cracked pepper	5	60	10	½	1	2	0.0	0	115	0
wheat	5	70	11	1	1	2	0.0	0	160	0
Sociables®	7	80	9	½	1	4	0.5	0	150	0
Table Water®	5	70	13	1	2	2	0.0	0	100	0
Teddy Grahams®	24	130	23	1½	2	4	0.5	0	140	0
Toasteds®, wheat										
reduced fat	5	60	10	½	1	2	0.0	0	160	0
regular	5	80	11	1	1	3	0.5	0	160	0
Triscuit®	7	140	21	1½	3	5	1.0	0	170	4
Valley Lahvosh™	4 (2 in.)	110	22	1½	4	1	0.0	0	150	0
Vegetable Thins®	14	160	19	1	2	9	1.5	0	310	1
Wasa®	1	45	9	½	1	0	0.0	0	40	2
Waverly®	5	70	10	½	1	4	0.5	0	135	0
Wheat Thins®										
low sodium	16	140	20	1	2	6	1.0	0	75	1

CRACKERS, DIPS & SNACK FOODS
Crackers

ITEM	AMOUNT	CALORIES	CARBOHYDRATE (g)	CARBOHYDRATE CHOICES	PROTEIN (g)	FAT (g)	SATURATED FAT (g)	CHOLESTEROL (mg)	SODIUM (mg)	FIBER (g)
Wheat Thins® *(con't.)*										
regular	16	140	19	1	2	6	1.0	0	180	2
Dips										
Bean	2 T.	40	5	0	2	1	0.0	0	170	1
Caramel apple	2 T.	160	23	1½	1	7	2.0	5	95	0
Cheese	2 T.	100	3	0	5	7	4.0	25	440	0
Dill	2 T.	100	2	0	1	10	4.0	10	170	0
French onion	2 T.	60	4	0	1	4	3.0	0	230	0
Fruit, w/ marshmallow creme	2 T.	90	11	1	0	5	4.0	5	55	0
Salsa, w/ cheese	2 T.	40	5	0	1	2	0.5	0	650	0
Spinach	2 T.	90	2	0	1	9	3.0	10	135	0
Snack Foods										
Bagel chips	5	60	9	½	2	3	0.5	0	180	2
Bugles®										
baked	1½ cups	130	22	1½	2	4	0.5	0	440	1
regular	1⅓ cups	160	18	1	1	9	8.0	0	310	1
Chee-tos®, crunchy	21	160	15	1	2	10	2.5	0	290	0
Cheez Balls, Planters®	34	160	15	1	2	10	2.5	0	300	0
Chex Mix®	⅔ cup	130	21	1½	3	4	0.5	0	410	1
Combos®, w/ cheddar	⅓ cup	130	19	1	3	5	1.0	0	300	1
Cornnuts®	⅓ cup	130	20	1	2	4	1.0	0	190	2
Cracker Jack®	1 cup	170	34	2	3	3	0.0	0	125	2
Doritos® nacho chips										
3Ds®	27	140	17	1	2	7	1.5	0	360	1
fat free	11	90	18	1	2	1	0.0	0	240	1
regular	11	140	17	1	2	7	1.5	0	200	1
Fritos®	32	160	15	1	2	10	1.5	0	170	1
Funyuns®	13	140	18	1	2	7	1.5	0	270	0
Popcorn										
air popped	3 cups	90	22	1½	3	2	0.0	0	1	3
caramel	1 cup	152	28	2	1	5	1.0	5	218	2
cheddar cheese	3 cups	190	17	1	3	13	2.5	0	300	3
oil popped, salted	3 cups	165	19	1	3	9	1.5	0	292	3
toffee, fat free	¾ cup	110	26	2	0	0	0.0	0	190	0
Popcorn, microwave										
butter	3 cups	105	12	1	2	8	2.0	0	180	3
Healthy Choice®	3 cups	50	11	1	2	1	0.0	0	70	3
light	3 cups	60	12	1	2	3	0.0	0	135	3
Popcorn cakes	1 (4 in.)	40	10	½	0	0	0.0	0	20	1
Pork rinds	28	155	0	0	17	9	3.0	27	521	0
Potato chips										
baked	11	120	22	1½	2	3	0.0	0	210	2

CRACKERS, DIPS & SNACK FOODS
Snack Foods

ITEM	AMOUNT	CALORIES	CARBOHYDRATE (g)	CARBOHYDRATE CHOICES	PROTEIN (g)	FAT (g)	SATURATED FAT (g)	CHOLESTEROL (mg)	SODIUM (mg)	FIBER (g)
Potato chips *(con't.)*										
BBQ	20	200	20	1	3	13	4.0	0	266	1
fat free	20	75	18	1	2	0	0.0	0	200	1
regular	20	150	15	1	2	10	3.0	0	180	1
Potato sticks	¾ cup	180	17	1	2	11	3.0	0	115	1
Pretzels										
Air Crisps®	23	110	23	1½	2	0	0.0	0	550	0
sourdough, hard	1	100	22	1½	3	0	0.0	0	240	1
toffee covered	12	120	25	1½	1	1	0.0	0	200	0
twists, large	9	110	23	1½	2	1	0.0	0	560	1
twists, small	17	110	23	1½	2	1	0.0	0	580	1
yogurt covered, small	7	140	21	1½	2	6	5.0	0	150	0
Pringles® potato crisps										
fat free	16	70	15	1	1	0	0.0	0	160	1
regular	12	160	14	1	2	10	2.5	0	180	1
Rice cakes										
mini, caramel	7 (2 in.)	60	13	1	1	0	0.0	0	150	0
regular, plain	2 (4 in.)	70	15	1	1	0	0.0	0	5	1
Sesame sticks	8	130	19	1	3	5	0.5	0	360	1
Sun Chips®	11	140	20	1	1	6	1.0	0	115	2
Tostitos® tortilla chips										
baked, bite size	20	110	24	1½	3	1	0.0	0	200	2
crispy rounds	13	150	17	1	2	8	1.0	0	85	1
restaurant style	6	130	19	1	2	6	1.0	0	80	1
restaurant style, fat free	6	90	20	1	2	1	0.0	0	105	1
Veggie Stix™	1 oz.	140	19	1	1	6	0.5	0	310	1
Wheat Nuts®	¼ cup	152	4	0	3	14	2.0	0	144	1

DESSERTS, SWEETS & TOPPINGS
Bars

ITEM	AMOUNT	CALORIES	CARBOHYDRATE (g)	CARBOHYDRATE CHOICES	PROTEIN (g)	FAT (g)	SATURATED FAT (g)	CHOLESTEROL (mg)	SODIUM (mg)	FIBER (g)
Brownies, butterscotch	1 (2 in.)	249	36	2½	3	11	2.0	29	159	0
Brownies, chocolate										
fat free	1 (2 in.)	120	28	2	1	0	0.0	0	180	0
regular, w/ nuts	1 (2 in.)	247	39	2½	3	10	2.5	10	190	1
regular, w/o nuts	1 (2 in.)	243	39	2½	3	10	3.0	10	153	0
Golden Grahams Treats™	1 (1 oz.)	90	17	1	1	3	0.5	0	100	0
Granola, plain	1 (1 oz.)	134	18	1	3	6	1.0	0	84	2
Kudos®, peanut butter	1 (1 oz.)	130	19	1	2	5	2.0	0	85	1
Lemon	1 (2 oz.)	250	46	3	3	6	1.5	50	150	1
Nutri-Grain Bar®	1 (1.3 oz.)	140	27	2	2	3	0.5	0	110	1
Nutty Bars®	1 (1 oz.)	155	16	1	3	9	1.5	0	55	1
Power Bar®	1 (2.3 oz.)	230	45	3	10	3	0.5	0	110	3

DESSERTS, SWEETS & TOPPINGS
Bars

ITEM	AMOUNT	CALORIES	CARBOHYDRATE (g)	CARBOHYDRATE CHOICES	PROTEIN (g)	FAT (g)	SATURATED FAT (g)	CHOLESTEROL (mg)	SODIUM (mg)	FIBER (g)
Rice Krispies Treats™	1 (0.8 oz.)	90	18	1	1	2	0.5	0	100	0
Seven layer	1 (2 in.)	271	33	2	3	15	10.5	16	115	1
Cakes, Pastries & Sweet Breads										
Angel food cake	½ cake	137	29	2	3	0	0.0	0	255	0
Apple dumplings	1 (5 oz.)	357	53	3½	2	16	3.5	0	302	2
Apple fritters	1 (1 oz.)	87	8	½	1	6	1.5	21	10	0
Baklava	1 (2 in.)	333	29	2	5	23	9.5	35	291	2
Banana bread	1 (2 in.)	185	31	2	2	6	1.0	24	171	1
Black forest cake	½ cake	280	32	2	3	15	3.0	46	224	1
Caramel rolls	1 (3.5 oz.)	320	52	3½	5	10	2.5	0	700	1
Carrot cake, iced	1 (4 oz.)	484	52	3½	5	29	5.0	60	273	1
Cheesecake										
plain	1 (3 oz.)	295	23	1½	5	21	11.0	51	190	0
Smart One's™	1 (2.5 oz.)	150	21	1½	6	5	2.5	15	140	1
turtle	1 (2.5 oz.)	270	19	1	4	21	12.0	65	80	2
Chocolate cake, iced	½ cake	253	38	2½	3	11	3.0	32	230	2
Cinnamon rolls	1 (3.5 oz.)	300	54	3½	5	7	2.0	0	720	1
Cobblers, fruit	1 (3 in.)	204	36	2½	2	6	1.0	1	291	2
Coffeecake										
cinnamon, w/ topping	1 (2 oz.)	240	30	2	4	12	2.0	36	233	1
fruit	1 (2 oz.)	176	29	2	3	6	1.5	4	218	1
Cream puffs	1 (4 oz.)	297	27	2	7	18	4.5	144	382	1
Crêpes, fruit filled	1 (4 oz.)	191	30	2	5	6	2.0	92	181	1
Crisps, fruit	1 (3 in.)	146	24	1½	2	5	1.0	0	74	1
Cupcakes, iced										
light	1 (1.5 oz.)	140	29	2	2	2	0.5	0	190	1
regular	1 (1.5 oz.)	180	30	2	2	6	2.5	5	290	1
Danish										
cheese	1 (2.5 oz.)	266	26	2	6	16	5.0	11	320	1
fruit	1 (2.5 oz.)	252	34	2	4	12	2.5	14	251	1
Ding Dongs™	1 (1.3 oz.)	190	23	1½	2	10	6.0	8	125	1
Doughnuts										
cake, plain	1 medium	198	23	1½	2	11	2.0	17	257	1
holes, glazed	5 medium	260	32	2	3	14	3.0	10	330	1
raised, glazed	1 medium	242	27	2	4	14	3.5	4	205	1
Éclairs, chocolate	1 (3 oz.)	246	23	1½	6	15	4.0	119	317	1
Funnel cake	1 (6 in.)	285	29	2	7	15	4.0	66	236	1
Gingerbread cake	1 (2 in.)	263	36	2½	3	12	3.0	24	242	1
Ho Hos®	1 (1 oz.)	130	17	1	1	6	4.0	10	75	1
Lemon cake, iced	1 (4 oz.)	404	73	5	3	12	2.5	35	258	1
Marble cake, iced	½ cake	404	59	4	3	19	4.5	53	311	1
Pineapple upside down cake	1 (2 in.)	367	58	4	4	14	3.5	25	367	1

DESSERTS, SWEETS & TOPPINGS
Cakes, Pastries & Sweet Breads

ITEM	AMOUNT	CALORIES	CARBOHYDRATE (g)	CARBOHYDRATE CHOICES	PROTEIN (g)	FAT (g)	SATURATED FAT (g)	CHOLESTEROL (mg)	SODIUM (mg)	FIBER (g)
Pop Tart®	1 (1.8 oz.)	204	37	2½	2	5	1.0	0	218	1
Pound cake	½₂ cake	206	29	2	3	9	2.0	41	172	0
Pumpkin bread	1 (2 in.)	188	29	2	2	7	1.0	25	177	1
Spice cake, iced	1 (4 oz.)	389	68	4½	4	12	4.0	50	282	1
Sponge cake	½₂ cake	110	23	1½	2	1	0.5	39	93	0
Strudel	1 (2 in.)	179	29	2	3	6	1.0	9	88	1
SuzyQ's®	1 (2 oz.)	230	35	2	2	9	4.0	10	270	1
Toaster Strudel™	1 (1.9 oz.)	180	27	2	3	7	1.5	6	202	1
Turnovers, fruit	1 (3 oz.)	289	36	2½	3	15	3.5	0	262	1
Twinkies®										
light	1 (1.5 oz.)	130	27	2	1	2	0.5	10	190	0
regular	1 (1.5 oz.)	150	25	1½	1	5	2.0	20	200	0
White cake, iced	½₂ cake	266	45	3	2	10	4.0	6	166	1
Yodels®	1 (1.1 oz.)	140	18	1	1	8	3.0	0	75	1
Cookies										
Biscotti										
almond	1	90	12	1	2	4	1.0	5	65	1
chocolate dipped	1	110	14	1	2	4	2.0	10	70	1
Chocolate chip										
Chips Ahoy®, reduced fat	1	47	7	½	1	2	0.5	0	50	0
Chips Ahoy®, regular	1	53	7	½	1	3	1.0	0	35	0
homemade	1 (2 in.)	78	9	½	1	5	1.5	5	58	0
Chocolate wafers	1	28	5	0	0	1	0.0	0	46	0
E. L. Fudge®	1	60	9	½	1	3	0.5	0	35	0
Fudge stripes	1	53	7	½	0	3	1.5	0	47	0
Ginger snaps	1	30	6	½	0	1	0.0	0	58	0
Girl Scout Cookies®										
Caramel deLites/Samoas®	1	70	10	½	1	4	3.0	0	43	1
Lemon Pastry Cremes	1	43	7	½	0	2	0.0	0	33	0
Peanut Butter Patties/Tagalongs®	1	75	8	½	1	4	2.5	0	58	1
Peanut Butter Sandwich/Do-si-dos	1	60	8	½	1	3	0.5	0	50	0
Thin Mints	1	40	5	0	0	2	1.5	0	35	0
Koala Yummies®	13	190	13	1	1	10	0.0	0	90	0
Lady fingers	1	40	7	½	1	1	0.5	40	16	0
Lido®	1	90	10	½	0	5	1.5	0	40	0
Lorna Doone®	1	35	5	0	1	2	0.5	1	33	0
Macaroons	1 (2 in.)	97	17	1	1	3	2.5	0	59	0
Milano®	1	57	7	½	1	3	1.0	3	37	0
Molasses	1	65	11	1	1	2	0.5	0	69	0
Monster	1 (5 in.)	565	72	4½	14	28	10.0	71	405	5
Newtons®, most varieties										
fat free	1	45	11	1	1	0	0.0	0	58	1

DESSERTS, SWEETS & TOPPINGS
Cookies

ITEM	AMOUNT	CALORIES	CARBOHYDRATE (g)	CARBOHYDRATE CHOICES	PROTEIN (g)	FAT (g)	SATURATED FAT (g)	CHOLESTEROL (mg)	SODIUM (mg)	FIBER (g)
Newtons®, most varieties *(con't.)*										
regular	1	55	11	1	1	1	0.0	0	58	1
Nutter Butter®	1	65	10	½	2	3	0.5	1	55	1
Oatmeal raisin	1	65	10	½	1	2	0.5	5	81	0
Oreo®										
double stuff	1	70	10	½	1	4	1.0	0	75	0
reduced fat	1	43	8	½	1	1	0.5	0	63	0
regular	1	54	8	½	1	3	0.5	0	74	1
Peanut butter	1	95	12	1	2	5	1.0	6	104	0
Pecan Sandies®	1	80	9	½	0	5	1.0	0	75	0
Sandwich										
fructose-sweetened	1	53	5	0	0	0	0.0	0	12	0
regular	1	48	7	½	0	2	0.5	0	35	0
Shortbread	1	60	6	½	1	4	2.5	10	51	0
SnackWell's®										
chocolate	1	55	10	½	0	2	0.5	0	35	0
chocolate chip, bite size	13	130	22	1½	2	4	1.5	0	160	0
mint creme	1	55	10	½	1	2	0.5	0	35	0
Social Tea® biscuits	1	20	4	0	0	1	0.0	1	19	0
Sugar	1	72	10	½	1	3	1.0	8	54	0
Sugar wafers	1	43	6	½	0	2	0.5	0	7	0
Vanilla wafers										
reduced fat	1	18	3	0	0	1	0.0	0	13	0
regular	1	15	3	0	0	0	0.0	0	13	0
Vienna Fingers®	1	70	11	1	1	3	1.0	0	53	0
Frozen Yogurt & Ice Cream										
Frozen yogurt										
fat free	½ cup	95	19	1	5	0	0.0	2	64	0
regular	½ cup	120	22	1½	3	3	2.0	10	55	0
Gelato	½ cup	130	23	1½	4	3	1.5	5	60	0
Ice cream										
fat free	½ cup	90	19	1	4	0	0.0	0	50	0
fat free, no added sugar	½ cup	70	17	1	3	0	0.0	0	55	0
light	½ cup	100	17	1	3	3	2.0	10	50	0
premium	½ cup	260	32	2	4	13	7.0	50	80	0
regular	½ cup	140	17	1	2	7	5.0	30	50	0
Sherbet	½ cup	132	29	2	1	2	1.0	5	44	0
Sorbet	½ cup	110	27	2	0	0	0.0	0	15	0
Ice Cream Novelties										
Baby Ruth® bars	1 (2.5 oz.)	180	15	1	3	12	7.0	10	35	0
Chipwich®	1 (3.3 oz.)	240	35	2	0	10	5.0	20	135	0
Chocolate éclair bars	1 (3 oz.)	170	21	1½	2	9	2.5	10	60	1

DESSERTS, SWEETS & TOPPINGS
Ice Cream Novelties

ITEM	AMOUNT	CALORIES	CARBOHYDRATE (g)	CARBOHYDRATE CHOICES	PROTEIN (g)	FAT (g)	SATURATED FAT (g)	CHOLESTEROL (mg)	SODIUM (mg)	FIBER (g)
Creamsicle®	1 (1.8 oz.)	80	14	1	0	2	1.5	5	20	0
Crunch® bars	1 (3 oz.)	200	19	1	2	13	10.0	20	50	0
Dove bar®	1 (3 oz.)	280	23	1½	5	19	11.0	30	110	1
Dove® bite size	5 (0.6 oz.)	330	33	2	3	21	13.0	50	35	0
Drumstick® cones	1 (4.6 oz.)	340	35	2	6	19	11.0	20	90	2
Eskimo Pie®	1 (2.5 oz.)	160	13	1	2	12	9.0	15	35	0
Frappuccino® bars	1 (2.5 oz.)	120	21	1½	4	2	1.0	10	50	0
Frozen yogurt bars	1 (2.4 oz.)	90	20	1	2	0	0.0	0	15	0
Fruit juice bars	1 (3 oz.)	63	16	1	1	0	0.0	0	3	0
Fudgsicle®										
no sugar added	1 (1.75 oz.)	45	9	½	1	1	0.0	0	45	0
regular	1 (1.75 oz.)	60	12	1	2	1	0.5	0	40	0
Heath® bars	1 (2.5 oz.)	170	15	1	2	12	9.0	20	40	0
Ice cream cone, cone only										
cake/wafer	1 (0.14 oz.)	17	3	0	0	0	0.0	0	6	0
sugar	1 (0.35 oz.)	40	8	½	1	0	0.0	0	32	0
waffle	1 (1.25 oz.)	160	29	2	3	4	1.0	5	70	0
Ice cream sandwiches	1 (2 oz.)	144	22	1½	3	6	3.0	20	36	1
Italian ice	½ cup	61	16	1	0	0	0.0	0	5	0
Klondike® bars	1 (5 oz.)	290	25	1½	4	20	14.0	30	70	0
M&M's® sandwiches	1 (2.7 oz.)	240	32	2	3	12	5.0	25	160	0
Popsicle®										
regular	1 (1.8 oz.)	45	11	1	0	0	0.0	0	0	0
sugar free	1 (1.8 oz.)	15	3	0	0	0	0.0	0	0	0
Pudding bars	1 (1.8 oz.)	80	15	1	3	2	1.0	5	65	0
Pushups, sherbet	1 (2.8 oz.)	100	20	1	1	2	1.0	5	25	0
Reese's™ ice cream cups	1 (2.1 oz.)	160	14	1	2	11	6.0	10	45	0
Rice Dream®										
mocha/vanilla pie	1 (3.8 oz.)	290	37	2½	3	15	7.0	0	70	2
nondairy dessert	½ cup	150	23	1½	0	6	0.5	0	100	1
Snickers® bars	1 (2 oz.)	180	18	1	3	11	6.0	10	60	0
Snow cones	1 (6.7 oz.)	148	62	4	1	0	0.0	0	42	0
Starbucks Coffee® bars	1 (3 oz.)	280	25	1½	4	18	9.0	25	45	1
Strawberry shortcake bars	1 (3 oz.)	160	23	1½	2	7	3.0	10	55	0
Tofutti®	½ cup	190	20	1	2	11	2.0	0	210	0
Vienetta®	1 slice	190	19	1	3	11	7.0	40	40	0
Ice Cream Toppings										
Butterscotch/caramel	2 T.	103	27	2	1	0	0.0	0	143	0
Hot fudge										
fat free	2 T.	100	25	1½	1	0	0.0	0	80	0
regular	2 T.	147	25	1½	2	5	2.5	5	55	1

DESSERTS, SWEETS & TOPPINGS
Pies

ITEM	AMOUNT	CALORIES	CARBOHYDRATE (g)	CARBOHYDRATE CHOICES	PROTEIN (g)	FAT (g)	SATURATED FAT (g)	CHOLESTEROL (mg)	SODIUM (mg)	FIBER (g)
Other Sweets										
Caramel apples	1 medium	255	56	4	2	4	3.0	3	111	4
Chocolate mousse										
homemade	½ cup	446	33	2	9	33	18.5	299	87	1
mix	½ cup	145	20	1	5	6	4.0	9	73	1
Crêpes Suzette, w/ sauce	1 (2.5 oz.)	173	17	1	4	10	4.5	90	175	0
Custard	½ cup	148	15	1	7	7	3.5	123	109	0
Flan, w/ caramel	½ cup	220	35	2	7	6	3.0	141	86	0
Gelatin										
regular	½ cup	80	19	1	2	0	0.0	0	57	0
sugar free	½ cup	8	1	0	1	0	0.0	0	56	0
Marshmallows	3 large	68	17	1	0	0	0.0	0	10	0
Pudding										
bread, hmde.	½ cup	212	31	2	7	7	3.0	83	291	1
chocolate, fat free	½ cup	100	23	1½	3	0	0.0	0	220	0
chocolate, instant, w/ 1%	½ cup	149	28	2	5	3	1.5	9	418	0
chocolate, regular, w/ 1%	½ cup	141	28	2	5	2	1.0	5	172	0
rice, hmde.	½ cup	217	40	2½	5	4	2.5	17	85	1
vanilla, sugar free, w/ 1%	½ cup	81	13	1	5	2	1.0	5	172	0
Pies										
Apple/cherry	⅛ pie	310	45	3	3	14	2.5	0	380	1
Banana cream	⅛ pie	387	47	3	6	20	5.5	73	346	1
Blueberry	⅛ pie	277	42	3	2	12	2.0	0	341	1
Boston cream	⅛ pie	232	39	2½	2	8	2.5	34	132	1
Coconut cream	⅛ pie	396	45	3	6	21	8.0	77	356	1
French silk	⅛ pie	420	55	3½	3	22	6.0	5	260	1
Grasshopper	⅛ pie	331	33	2	5	18	6.0	98	476	0
Hostess® fruit	1 (4.5 oz.)	470	65	4	3	22	11.0	20	470	1
Lemon meringue	⅛ pie	362	50	3	5	16	4.0	67	307	2
Pecan	⅛ pie	503	64	4	6	27	5.0	106	320	4
Pumpkin	⅛ pie	260	34	2	3	13	3.0	55	210	1
Rhubarb	⅛ pie	299	45	3	3	13	3.0	0	319	1
Shoo fly	⅛ pie	397	67	4½	4	13	3.0	37	208	1
Strawberry chiffon	⅛ pie	331	41	3	4	17	8.0	35	204	2
Sweet potato	⅛ pie	319	35	2	6	17	5.0	66	197	2
Syrups & Toppings										
Apple butter	1 T.	31	8	½	0	0	0.0	0	1	0
Artificial sweeteners										
Equal®	¼ tsp.	0	0	0	0	0	0.0	0	0	0
Sugar Twin®	1 tsp.	0	0	0	0	0	0.0	0	0	0
Sweet 'N Low®	⅒ tsp.	0	0	0	0	0	0.0	0	0	0

DESSERTS, SWEETS & TOPPINGS
Syrups & Toppings

ITEM	AMOUNT	CALORIES	CARBOHYDRATE (g)	CARBOHYDRATE CHOICES	PROTEIN (g)	FAT (g)	SATURATED FAT (g)	CHOLESTEROL (mg)	SODIUM (mg)	FIBER (g)
Chocolate syrup										
lite	2 T.	50	12	1	0	0	0.0	0	35	0
regular	2 T.	100	24	1½	1	0	0.0	0	25	0
Coffee syrup	1 T.	40	11	1	0	0	0.0	0	0	0
Frosting/icing										
chocolate	2 T.	138	27	2	0	4	2.5	10	65	1
reduced fat	2 T.	120	24	1½	0	2	1.0	0	75	0
vanilla	2 T.	137	31	2	0	2	1.0	5	26	0
Fruit spread	1 T.	20	5	0	0	0	0.0	0	20	0
Grenadine syrup	1 tsp.	18	5	0	0	0	0.0	0	3	0
Honey	1 tsp.	21	6	½	0	0	0.0	0	0	0
Jam/jelly/marmalade	1 T.	48	13	1	0	0	0.0	0	8	0
Maple syrup	1 T.	52	13	1	0	0	0.0	0	2	0
Marshmallow creme	2 T.	60	15	1	0	0	0.0	0	10	0
Pancake syrup										
low calorie	1 T.	23	6	½	0	0	0.0	0	28	0
regular	1 T.	56	15	1	0	0	0.0	0	16	0
Sugar, brown/raw/white	1 tsp.	16	4	0	0	0	0.0	0	0	0
Whipped cream, hmde.	2 T.	58	2	0	0	6	4.0	20	6	0
Whipped toppings										
Cool-Whip®, Free™	2 T.	15	3	0	0	0	0.0	0	5	0
Cool-Whip®, Lite®	2 T.	20	2	0	0	1	1.0	0	0	0
Cool-Whip®, regular	2 T.	25	2	0	0	2	1.5	0	0	0
Reddi Wip®	2 T.	20	0	0	0	2	1.0	5	0	0
sugar free, mix	2 T.	10	1	0	0	1	0.0	0	5	0
EGGS, EGG DISHES & EGG SUBSTITUTES										
Eggs										
Chicken										
boiled/poached	1 large	75	1	0	6	5	1.5	213	63	0
deviled, w/ filling	½ large	63	0	0	4	5	1.0	121	94	0
fried, w/ ½ tsp. fat	1 large	92	1	0	6	7	2.0	211	162	0
scrambled, w/ 1 tsp. fat	2 large	203	3	0	14	15	4.5	429	342	0
whites	2	33	1	0	7	0	0.0	0	212	0
yolk	1	59	0	0	3	5	1.5	212	33	0
Duck	1	130	1	0	9	10	2.5	619	102	0
Goose	1	266	2	0	20	19	5.0	1227	199	0
Quail	1	14	0	0	1	1	0.0	76	13	0
Turkey	1	135	1	0	11	9	3.0	737	119	0
Egg Dishes										
Frittatas, 10 in.	⅙ pie	233	8	½	16	15	5.0	429	262	0

EGGS, EGG DISHES & EGG SUBSTITUTES
Egg Dishes

ITEM	AMOUNT	CALORIES	CARBOHYDRATE (g)	CARBOHYDRATE CHOICES	PROTEIN (g)	FAT (g)	SATURATED FAT (g)	CHOLESTEROL (mg)	SODIUM (mg)	FIBER (g)
Omelets										
ham & cheese	1 (3 egg)	274	2	0	21	19	6.0	605	478	0
vegetable	1 (3 egg)	213	3	0	17	14	4.0	560	165	1
Quiche										
cheese	4 oz.	344	15	1	10	28	13.5	142	254	0
Lorraine	4 oz.	321	13	1	10	26	12.0	127	253	0
spinach	4 oz.	266	13	1	9	20	9.5	122	258	1
Soufflés										
cheese	1 cup	197	6	½	12	14	6.0	194	298	0
spinach	1 cup	219	3	0	11	18	7.0	184	763	3
Egg Substitutes										
Egg Beaters®	¼ cup	30	1	0	6	0	0.0	0	100	0
Powdered	1½ tsp.	15	4	0	0	0	0.0	0	5	0
Second Nature®	¼ cup	30	1	0	7	0	0.0	0	110	0

FAST FOODS
Arby's®

ITEM	AMOUNT	CALORIES	CARBOHYDRATE (g)	CARBOHYDRATE CHOICES	PROTEIN (g)	FAT (g)	SATURATED FAT (g)	CHOLESTEROL (mg)	SODIUM (mg)	FIBER (g)
Baked potatoes										
broccoli 'n cheddar	1	550	71	4	14	25	13.0	50	730	7
chicken broccoli	1	830	68	4	35	47	8.0	60	970	7
chicken Philly	1	880	75	4½	32	53	10.0	70	1020	7
cool ranch	1	500	67	4	8	23	7.0	25	150	6
deluxe	1	610	68	4	14	31	19.0	80	860	6
jalapeño	1	660	72	4½	15	36	14.0	50	930	6
plain	1	270	63	4	6	0	0.0	0	20	6
w/ butter & sour cream	1	500	65	4	8	24	15.0	60	170	6
Biscuit, w/ butter	1	269	26	2	5	16	3.0	0	750	0
Chicken finger meal	1 order	880	81	5½	35	47	8.0	60	2240	0
Chicken finger snack	1 order	610	62	4	20	32	6.0	30	1610	0
Chicken fingers	2	270	19	1	15	15	2.0	30	630	0
Chicken sandwiches										
bacon & Swiss	1	610	52	3	37	30	9.0	75	1620	5
breaded fillet	1	560	49	3	30	28	6.0	50	1080	6
cordon bleu	1	650	50	3	40	34	9.0	90	2120	5
grilled deluxe	1	420	42	3	30	16	4.0	60	930	3
light grilled	1	280	33	2	30	5	1.5	50	920	4
light roast deluxe	1	260	32	2	24	5	1.5	40	950	4
roast club	1	540	39	2½	37	29	8.0	70	1590	3
spicy	1	520	50	3	27	25	4.0	40	1030	2
Croissants										
bacon & egg	1	570	29	2	16	31	14.0	170	780	0
ham & cheese	1	400	29	2	18	25	14.0	55	720	0

FAST FOODS

Arby's®

ITEM	AMOUNT	CALORIES	CARBOHYDRATE (g)	CARBOHYDRATE CHOICES	PROTEIN (g)	FAT (g)	SATURATED FAT (g)	CHOLESTEROL (mg)	SODIUM (mg)	FIBER (g)
Croissants *(con't.)*										
plain	1	260	28	2	6	16	10.0	22	300	0
Curly fries										
regular	medium	380	49	3	5	19	4.5	0	1100	0
w/ cheddar	medium	450	52	3½	7	25	6.0	5	1420	0
Dipping sauces										
Bronco Berry™	1 pkt.	90	23	1½	0	0	0.0	0	35	0
Horsey Sauce®	1 pkt.	60	2	0	0	5	1.0	5	150	0
marinara	1 pkt.	35	4	0	1	2	0.0	0	260	0
Tangy Southwest™	1 pkt.	250	25	1½	0	25	4.0	30	280	0
Fish fillet	1	540	51	3½	23	27	7.0	40	880	2
French fries	medium	420	57	4	5	19	3.0	0	830	4
French-toastix	1 order	370	48	3	7	17	4.0	0	440	4
Hot ham 'n Swiss sub	1	570	47	3	30	31	10.0	100	2560	2
Italian sub	1	800	49	3	28	54	16.0	85	2610	2
Jalapeño Bites™	1 order	330	29	2	7	21	9.0	40	670	2
Mozzarella sticks	1 order	470	34	2	18	29	14.0	60	1330	2
Onion petals	1 order	410	43	3	4	24	3.0	0	300	2
Potato cakes	2	220	21	1½	2	14	3.0	0	460	3
Roast beef sandwiches										
Arby-Q®	1	380	42	3	19	15	5.0	30	990	3
Arby's melt, w/ cheddar	1	380	38	2½	19	19	7.0	31	960	3
beef 'n cheddar	1	510	45	3	26	28	9.0	50	1250	3
Big Montana®	1	720	44	2½	50	40	17.0	110	2270	7
French dip sub	1	490	43	3	30	22	8.0	55	1440	3
giant	1	550	43	2½	34	28	11.0	70	1560	5
junior	1	340	36	2½	18	16	6.0	30	790	3
Philly beef 'n Swiss sub	1	780	52	3½	39	48	16.0	90	2140	4
regular	1	400	36	2½	23	20	7.0	40	1030	4
super	1	530	50	3	24	27	9.0	40	1190	5
Salad dressings										
blue cheese	1 pkt.	290	2	0	2	31	6.0	50	580	0
honey French	1 pkt.	280	18	1	0	23	3.0	0	400	0
Italian, reduced calorie	1 pkt.	20	3	0	0	1	0.0	0	1000	0
Salads, w/o dressing, w/ crackers & croutons										
light garden	1	200	30	2	11	5	1.0	0	410	1
light grilled chicken	1	280	31	2	27	7	1.0	40	790	1
light roast chicken	1	290	31	2	27	7	1.0	40	1060	1
light side	1	170	26	2	8	6	1.0	0	390	1
Shakes										
chocolate	16 fl. oz.	380	66	4½	8	9	6.0	10	300	0

FAST FOODS

Arby's®

ITEM	AMOUNT	CALORIES	CARBOHYDRATE (g)	CARBOHYDRATE CHOICES	PROTEIN (g)	FAT (g)	SATURATED FAT (g)	CHOLESTEROL (mg)	SODIUM (mg)	FIBER (g)
Shakes *(con't.)*										
jamocha	16 fl. oz.	390	69	4½	8	9	6.0	10	270	0
strawberry	16 fl. oz.	380	67	4½	8	9	6.0	10	270	0
vanilla	16 fl. oz.	380	67	4½	8	9	6.0	10	270	0
Turkey sandwiches										
light roast deluxe	1	230	33	2	19	5	1.5	25	870	4
sub	1	670	49	3	29	39	10.0	60	2130	2
Turnovers										
apple	1	340	49	3	4	14	3.0	0	180	0
cherry	1	330	47	3	4	13	3.0	0	190	0
Burger King®										
Biscuits										
plain	1	300	35	2	6	15	3.0	0	830	1
w/ egg	1	380	37	2½	11	21	5.0	140	1010	0
w/ sausage	1	490	36	2½	13	33	10.0	35	1240	1
w/ sausage, egg & cheese	1	620	37	2½	20	43	14.0	185	1650	1
BK Big Fish® sandwich	1	720	59	4	23	43	9.0	80	1180	3
Chicken sandwiches										
BK Broiler®	1	530	45	3	29	26	5.0	105	1060	2
w/o mayo.	1	370	45	3	29	9	5.0	105	1060	2
chicken sandwich	1	710	54	3½	26	43	9.0	60	1400	2
w/o mayo.	1	500	54	3½	26	20	9.0	60	1400	2
Chick'n crisp	1	460	37	2½	16	27	6.0	35	890	3
w/o mayo.	1	360	37	2½	16	16	6.0	35	890	3
Chicken Tenders®	4	180	9	½	11	11	3.0	30	470	0
Cini-minis, w/o icing	4	440	51	3½	6	23	6.0	25	710	1
Croissan'wich®										
sausage & cheese	1	450	21	1½	13	35	12.0	45	940	1
sausage, egg & cheese	1	530	23	1½	18	41	13.0	185	1120	1
Dutch apple pie	1	300	39	2½	3	15	3.0	0	230	2
French fries										
small, salted	1 order	250	32	2	2	13	5.0	0	550	2
small, unsalted	1 order	250	32	2	2	13	5.0	0	480	2
medium, salted	1 order	400	50	3	3	21	8.0	0	820	4
medium, unsalted	1 order	400	50	3	3	21	8.0	0	760	4
king size, salted	1 order	590	74	4½	5	30	12.0	0	1180	5
French toast sticks, w/o syrup	5	440	51	3½	7	23	5.0	2	490	3
Hamburgers										
bacon cheeseburger	1	400	27	2	24	22	10.0	70	940	1
bacon double cheeseburger	1	620	28	2	41	38	18.0	125	1230	1
Big King™	1	640	28	2	38	42	18.0	125	980	1
cheeseburger	1	360	27	2	21	19	9.0	60	760	1

FAST FOODS
Burger King®

ITEM	AMOUNT	CALORIES	CARBOHYDRATE (g)	CARBOHYDRATE CHOICES	PROTEIN (g)	FAT (g)	SATURATED FAT (g)	CHOLESTEROL (mg)	SODIUM (mg)	FIBER (g)
Hamburgers *(con't.)*										
double cheeseburger	1	580	27	2	38	36	17.0	120	1060	1
Double Whopper®	1	920	47	3	49	59	21.0	155	980	3
w/o mayo.	1	760	47	3	49	42	21.0	155	980	3
Double Whopper®, w/ cheese	1	1010	47	3	55	67	26.0	180	1460	3
w/o mayo.	1	850	47	3	55	50	26.0	180	1460	3
hamburger	1	320	27	2	19	15	6.0	50	520	1
Whopper®	1	660	47	3	29	40	12.0	85	900	3
w/o mayo.	1	510	47	3	29	23	12.0	85	900	3
Whopper®, w/ cheese	1	760	47	3	35	48	17.0	110	1380	3
w/o mayo.	1	600	47	3	35	31	17.0	110	1380	3
Whopper Jr.®	1	400	28	2	19	24	8.0	55	530	2
w/o mayo.	1	320	28	2	19	15	8.0	55	530	2
Whopper Jr.®, w/ cheese	1	450	28	2	22	28	10.0	65	770	2
w/o mayo.	1	370	28	2	22	19	10.0	65	770	2
Hash brown rounds	small	240	25	1½	2	15	6.0	0	440	2
Onion rings	medium	380	46	3	5	19	4.0	2	550	4
Shakes										
chocolate	medium	570	105	7	14	10	6.0	30	520	3
strawberry	medium	550	104	7	13	9	5.0	30	350	2
vanilla	medium	430	73	5	13	9	5.0	30	330	2
Value meals, king size,										
w/ king size drink & king size fries										
BK Big Fish™	1 meal	1717	235	15	28	73	21.0	80	2560	8
Double Whopper®	1 meal	1917	223	14	54	89	33.0	155	2360	8
Whopper®	1 meal	1657	223	14	34	70	24.0	85	2280	8
Value meals, regular,										
w/ medium drink & medium fries										
bacon double cheeseburger	1 meal	1300	148	9½	44	59	26.0	125	2188	5
Big King™	1 meal	1320	148	9½	41	63	26.0	125	1938	5
BK Big Fish®	1 meal	1400	179	11½	26	64	17.0	80	2138	7
chicken sandwich	1 meal	1390	174	11	29	64	17.0	60	2358	6
Double Whopper®	1 meal	1600	167	10½	52	80	29.0	155	1938	7
two cheeseburger	1 meal	1400	174	11	45	59	26.0	120	2478	6
Whopper®	1 meal	1340	167	10½	32	61	20.0	85	1858	7
Whopper Jr.®	1 meal	1080	148	9½	22	45	16.0	55	1488	6
Dairy Queen®										
Banana split	1	510	96	6½	8	12	8.0	30	180	3
Blizzard®, cookie dough										
small	1	660	99	6½	12	24	13.0	55	440	1
medium	1	950	143	9½	17	36	19.0	75	660	2

FAST FOODS
Dairy Queen®

ITEM	AMOUNT	CALORIES	CARBOHYDRATE (g)	CARBOHYDRATE CHOICES	PROTEIN (g)	FAT (g)	SATURATED FAT (g)	CHOLESTEROL (mg)	SODIUM (mg)	FIBER (g)
Blizzard®, sandwich cookie										
small	1	520	79	5	10	18	9.0	40	380	1
medium	1	640	97	6½	12	23	11.0	45	500	1
Breeze®, Heath®										
small	1	470	85	5½	11	10	6.0	10	380	1
medium	1	710	123	8	15	18	11.0	20	580	1
Breeze®, strawberry										
small	1	320	68	4½	10	1	0.5	5	190	1
medium	1	460	99	6½	13	1	1.0	10	270	1
Buster Bar®	1	450	41	3	10	28	12.0	15	280	2
Chicken sandwiches										
chicken breast fillet	1	430	37	2½	24	20	4.0	55	760	2
grilled chicken	1	310	30	2	24	10	2.5	50	1040	3
Chicken strip basket	1	1000	102	6½	35	50	13.0	55	2260	5
Chili 'n' cheese dog	1	330	22	1½	14	21	9.0	45	1090	2
Chocolate Dilly® bar	1	210	21	1½	3	13	7.0	10	75	0
Dipped cone										
small	1	340	42	3	6	17	9.0	20	130	1
medium	1	490	59	4	8	24	13.0	30	190	1
DQ® frzn. 8 in. cake	⅛ cake	340	53	3½	7	12	7.0	25	250	1
DQ® fudge bar	1	50	13	1	4	0	0.0	0	70	0
DQ Homestyle® burgers										
bacon double cheeseburger	1	610	31	2	41	36	18.0	130	1380	2
cheeseburger	1	340	29	2	20	17	8.0	55	850	2
double cheeseburger	1	540	30	2	35	31	16.0	115	1130	2
hamburger	1	290	29	2	17	12	5.0	45	630	2
Ultimate®	1	670	29	2	40	43	19.0	135	1210	2
DQ® ice cream sandwich	1	150	24	1½	3	5	2.0	5	115	1
DQ® soft serve, cone, chocolate										
small	1	240	37	2½	6	8	5.0	20	115	0
medium	1	340	53	3½	8	11	7.0	30	160	0
DQ® soft serve, cone, vanilla										
small	1	230	38	2½	6	7	4.5	20	115	0
medium	1	330	53	3½	8	9	6.0	30	160	0
large	1	410	65	4	10	12	8.0	40	200	0
DQ® soft serve, cup										
chocolate	½ cup	150	22	1½	4	5	3.5	15	75	0
vanilla	½ cup	140	22	1½	3	5	3.0	15	70	0
DQ® Treatzza Pizza®	⅛ pizza	180	28	2	3	7	3.5	5	160	1
DQ® vanilla orange bar	1	60	17	1	2	0	0.0	0	40	0
DQ® yogurt										
cone	medium	260	56	4	9	1	0.5	5	160	0

FAST FOODS

Dairy Queen®

ITEM	AMOUNT	CALORIES	CARBOHYDRATE (g)	CARBOHYDRATE CHOICES	PROTEIN (g)	FAT (g)	SATURATED FAT (g)	CHOLESTEROL (mg)	SODIUM (mg)	FIBER (g)
DQ® yogurt *(con't.)*										
cup	½ cup	100	21	1½	3	0	0.0	0	70	0
French fries	small	350	42	3	4	18	3.5	0	630	3
Fudge Cake Supreme™	1	890	124	8	11	38	22.0	65	960	3
Hot dog	1	240	19	1	9	14	5.0	25	730	1
Lemon DQ Freez'r®	½ cup	80	20	1	0	0	0.0	0	10	0
Malts, chocolate										
small	1	650	111	7½	15	16	10.0	55	370	0
medium	1	880	153	10	19	22	14.0	70	500	0
Misty® slush										
small	1	220	56	4	0	0	0.0	0	20	0
medium	1	290	74	5	0	0	0.0	0	30	0
Onion rings	1 order	320	39	2½	5	16	4.0	0	180	3
Peanut Buster® parfait	1	730	99	6½	16	31	17.0	35	400	2
Shakes										
small	1	560	94	6	13	15	10.0	50	310	0
medium	1	770	130	8½	17	20	13.0	70	420	0
Starkiss®	1	80	21	1½	0	0	0.0	0	10	0
Strawberry shortcake	1	430	70	4½	7	14	9.0	60	360	1
Sundaes, chocolate										
small	1	280	49	3	5	7	4.5	20	140	0
medium	1	400	71	5	8	10	6.0	30	210	0
Domino's Pizza®										
BBQ wings	1	50	2	0	6	2	1.0	26	175	0
Breadsticks	1	78	11	1	2	3	1.0	0	158	0
Cheese pizza										
deep dish, 6 in.	1 pizza	595	68	4½	23	27	11.0	24	1300	4
deep dish, 12 in.	1 slice	239	28	2	9	11	4.0	10	543	2
hand tossed	1 slice	174	25	1½	7	6	2.5	8	362	2
thin crust	¼ medium	271	31	2	12	12	5.0	15	809	2
Cheesy bread	1 piece	103	11	1	3	5	2.0	5	187	0
Extra cheese pizza										
deep dish, 12 in.	1 slice	263	28	2	11	13	6.0	13	618	2
hand tossed	1 slice	198	25	1½	9	7	4.0	11	437	2
thin crust	¼ medium	318	31	2	15	16	8.0	22	959	2
Garden salad	large	39	8	½	2	0	0.0	0	26	3
Ham pizza										
deep dish, 12 in.	1 slice	247	28	2	11	11	4.5	13	624	2
hand tossed	1 slice	183	25	1½	9	6	2.5	11	443	2
thin crust	¼ medium	288	31	2	14	12	5.0	22	972	2
Hot wings	1	45	1	0	5	2	1.0	26	354	0

FAST FOODS

Domino's Pizza®

ITEM	AMOUNT	CALORIES	CARBOHYDRATE (g)	CARBOHYDRATE CHOICES	PROTEIN (g)	FAT (g)	SATURATED FAT (g)	CHOLESTEROL (mg)	SODIUM (mg)	FIBER (g)
Pepperoni pizza										
deep dish, 6 in.	1 pizza	644	68	4½	25	32	12.0	34	1459	4
deep dish, 12 in.	1 slice	270	28	2	11	14	5.5	16	642	2
hand tossed	1 slice	205	25	1½	9	8	3.5	14	461	2
thin crust	¼ medium	333	31	2	15	17	7.0	28	1008	3
Sausage pizza										
deep dish, 6 in.	1 pizza	639	69	4½	25	31	12.0	33	1436	4
deep dish, 12 in.	1 slice	266	29	2	11	13	5.0	16	628	2
hand tossed	1 slice	201	26	2	9	8	3.5	13	447	2
thin crust	¼ medium	326	32	2	14	16	7.0	26	980	2
Veggie pizza										
deep dish, 12 in.	1 slice	257	29	2	10	12	4.5	10	707	2
hand tossed	1 slice	192	26	2	8	7	3.0	8	526	2
thin crust	¼ medium	307	34	2	13	15	6.0	15	1137	3
Hardee's®										
Apple turnover	1	270	38	2½	4	12	4.0	0	250	n/a
Biscuits										
Apple Cinnamon 'N' Raisin™	1	250	42	3	2	8	2.0	0	350	n/a
bacon, egg & cheese	1	520	45	3	17	30	11.0	210	1420	n/a
Biscuit 'N' Gravy™	1	530	56	4	10	30	9.0	15	1550	n/a
chicken	1	590	62	4	24	27	7.0	45	1820	n/a
country ham	1	440	44	3	14	22	7.0	30	1710	n/a
ham	1	410	45	3	13	20	6.0	25	1200	n/a
omelet	1	550	45	3	20	32	12.0	225	1350	n/a
plain	1	390	44	3	6	21	6.0	0	1000	n/a
sausage	1	550	44	3	12	36	11.0	25	1310	n/a
sausage & egg	1	620	45	3	19	41	13.0	225	1370	n/a
steak	1	580	56	4	15	32	10.0	30	1580	n/a
Chicken, fried										
breast	1	370	29	2	29	15	4.0	75	1190	n/a
leg	1	170	15	1	13	7	2.0	45	570	n/a
thigh	1	330	30	2	19	15	4.0	60	1000	n/a
wing	1	200	23	1½	10	8	2.0	30	740	n/a
Chicken sandwiches										
chicken fillet	1	480	44	3	24	23	4.0	55	1190	n/a
grilled chicken	1	350	28	2	23	16	3.0	65	860	n/a
Cole slaw	small	240	13	1	2	20	3.0	10	340	n/a
Crispy Curls™ potatoes	medium	340	41	3	5	18	4.0	0	950	n/a
Fisherman's Fillet™	1	530	45	3	25	28	7.0	75	1280	n/a
French fries										
regular	1 order	340	45	3	4	16	2.0	0	390	n/a
large	1 order	440	59	4	5	21	3.0	0	520	n/a

FAST FOODS

Hardee's®

ITEM	AMOUNT	CALORIES	CARBOHYDRATE (g)	CARBOHYDRATE CHOICES	PROTEIN (g)	FAT (g)	SATURATED FAT (g)	CHOLESTEROL (mg)	SODIUM (mg)	FIBER (g)
French fries *(con't.)*										
monster	1 order	510	67	4½	6	24	3.0	0	590	n/a
Frisco™ breakfast sandwich	1	450	42	3	22	22	8.0	225	1290	n/a
Gravy	1.5 oz.	20	3	0	0	0	0.0	0	260	n/a
Hamburgers										
bacon cheeseburger	1	720	42	3	30	48	15.0	105	1200	n/a
bacon double cheeseburger	1	1000	42	3	50	70	25.0	185	1575	n/a
Big Deluxe™	1	650	40	2½	24	44	11.0	75	870	n/a
cheeseburger	1	320	30	2	16	15	7.0	40	780	n/a
double cheeseburger	1	480	31	2	26	28	13.0	75	1055	n/a
Frisco™	1	720	37	2½	31	49	15.0	95	1180	n/a
hamburger	1	270	29	2	13	11	4.0	35	550	n/a
Monster Burger®	1	1060	37	2½	49	79	29.0	185	1860	n/a
Hash Rounds™	16	230	24	1½	3	14	3.0	0	560	n/a
Hot dog, w/ condiments	1	450	25	1½	15	32	12.0	55	1240	n/a
Hot Ham 'N' Cheese™	1	300	34	2	16	12	6.0	50	1390	n/a
Mashed potatoes	small	70	14	1	2	0	0.0	0	330	n/a
Peach cobbler	small	310	60	4	2	7	1.0	0	360	n/a
Roast beef sandwiches										
Big Roast Beef™	1	410	26	2	24	24	9.0	40	1140	n/a
regular	1	310	26	2	17	16	6.0	40	800	n/a
Shakes										
chocolate	small	370	67	4½	13	5	3.0	30	270	n/a
vanilla	small	350	65	4	12	5	3.0	20	300	n/a
Twist cone	1	180	34	2	4	2	1.0	10	120	n/a
KFC®										
BBQ baked beans	1 order	190	33	2	6	3	1.0	5	760	6
Biscuit	1	180	20	1	4	10	2.5	0	560	0
Chicken sandwiches										
BBQ	1	256	28	2	17	8	1.0	57	782	2
Original Recipe®	1	497	46	3	29	22	5.0	52	1213	3
Chunky chicken pot pie	1	770	69	4	29	42	13.0	70	2160	5
Cole slaw	1 order	180	21	1½	2	9	1.5	5	280	3
Colonel's Crispy Strips®	3	261	10	½	20	16	4.0	40	658	3
Corn on the cob	1 order	150	35	2	5	2	0.0	0	20	2
Cornbread	1 order	228	25	1½	3	13	2.0	42	194	1
Extra Tasty Crispy™ chicken										
breast	1	470	25	1½	31	28	7.0	80	930	1
drumstick	1	190	8	½	13	11	3.0	60	260	0
thigh	1	370	18	1	19	25	6.0	70	540	2
wing	1	200	10	½	10	13	4.0	45	290	0
Green beans	1 order	45	7	½	1	2	0.5	5	730	3

FAST FOODS

KFC

ITEM	AMOUNT	CALORIES	CARBOHYDRATE (g)	CARBOHYDRATE CHOICES	PROTEIN (g)	FAT (g)	SATURATED FAT (g)	CHOLESTEROL (mg)	SODIUM (mg)	FIBER (g)
Hot & spicy chicken										
breast	1	530	23	1½	32	35	8.0	110	1110	2
drumstick	1	190	10	½	13	11	3.0	50	300	0
thigh	1	370	13	1	18	27	7.0	90	570	1
wing	1	210	9	½	10	15	4.0	50	340	0
Hot Wings™	6	471	18	1	27	33	8.0	150	1230	2
Macaroni & cheese	1 order	180	21	1½	7	8	3.0	10	860	2
Mashed potatoes, w/ gravy	1 order	120	17	1	1	6	1.0	0	440	2
Mean Greens®	1 order	70	11	½	4	3	1.0	10	650	5
Original Recipe® chicken										
breast	1	400	16	1	29	24	6.0	135	1116	1
drumstick	1	140	4	0	13	9	2.0	75	422	0
thigh	1	250	6	½	16	18	4.5	95	747	1
wing	1	140	5	0	9	10	2.5	55	414	0
Potato salad	1 order	230	23	1½	4	14	2.0	15	540	3
Potato wedges	1 order	280	28	1½	5	13	4.0	5	750	5
Tender Roast® chicken										
breast	1	251	1	0	37	11	3.0	151	830	0
w/o skin	1	169	1	0	31	4	1.0	112	797	0
drumstick	1	97	0	0	15	4	1.0	85	271	0
w/o skin	1	67	0	0	11	2	0.5	63	259	0
thigh	1	207	1	0	18	12	4.0	120	504	0
w/o skin	1	106	0	0	13	6	1.5	84	312	0
wing	1	121	1	0	12	8	2.0	74	331	0
McDonald's®										
Apple bran muffin	1	300	61	4	6	3	0.5	0	380	3
Apple pie	1	260	34	2	3	13	3.5	0	200	0
Biscuits										
bacon, egg & cheese	1	470	36	2½	18	28	8.0	235	1250	1
plain	1	290	34	2	5	15	3.0	0	780	1
sausage	1	470	35	2	11	31	9.0	35	1080	1
sausage & egg	1	550	35	2	18	37	10.0	245	1160	1
Breakfast burrito	1	320	23	1½	13	20	7.0	195	600	2
Chicken McNuggets®										
4 piece	1 order	190	10	½	12	11	2.5	40	340	0
6 piece	1 order	290	15	1	18	17	3.5	60	510	0
Chicken sandwiches										
Crispy Chicken Deluxe™	1	500	43	3	26	25	4.0	55	1100	4
Grilled Chicken Deluxe™	1	440	38	2½	27	20	3.0	60	1040	4
w/o mayo.	1	300	38	2½	27	5	1.0	50	930	4
Cinnamon roll	1	390	50	3	6	18	5.0	65	310	2

FAST FOODS
McDonald's®

ITEM	AMOUNT	CALORIES	CARBOHYDRATE (g)	CARBOHYDRATE CHOICES	PROTEIN (g)	FAT (g)	SATURATED FAT (g)	CHOLESTEROL (mg)	SODIUM (mg)	FIBER (g)
Danish										
apple	1	360	51	3½	5	16	5.0	40	290	1
cheese	1	410	47	3	7	22	8.0	70	340	0
Egg McMuffin®	1	290	27	2	17	12	4.5	235	790	1
Filet-O-Fish®	1	450	42	3	16	25	4.5	50	870	2
Fish Filet Deluxe™	1	560	54	3½	23	28	6.0	60	1060	4
French fries										
small	1 order	210	26	2	3	10	1.5	0	135	2
large	1 order	450	57	3½	6	22	4.0	0	290	5
Super Size®	1 order	540	68	4	8	26	4.5	0	350	6
Hamburgers										
Arch Deluxe®	1	550	39	2½	28	31	11.0	90	1010	4
Arch Deluxe®, w/ bacon	1	590	39	2½	32	34	12.0	100	1150	4
Big Mac®	1	560	45	3	26	31	10.0	85	1070	3
cheeseburger	1	320	35	2	15	13	6.0	40	820	2
hamburger	1	260	34	2	13	9	3.5	30	580	2
Quarter Pounder®	1	420	37	2½	23	21	8.0	70	820	2
Quarter Pounder®, w/ cheese	1	530	38	2½	28	30	13.0	95	1290	2
Hash browns	1	130	14	1	1	8	1.5	0	330	1
Hot cakes, w/ marg. & syrup	1 order	610	104	7	9	18	3.5	25	680	2
Ice cream cone, vanilla	1	150	23	1½	4	5	3.0	20	75	0
McDonaldland® cookies	1 pkt.	180	32	2	3	5	1.0	0	190	1
McFlurry™										
Butterfinger®	1 (12 oz.)	620	90	6	16	22	14.0	70	260	0
M&M®	1 (12 oz.)	630	90	6	16	23	15.0	75	210	1
Nestle Crunch®	1 (12 oz.)	630	89	6	16	24	16.0	75	230	0
Oreo®	1 (12 oz.)	570	82	5½	15	20	12.0	70	280	0
Salad dressings										
Caesar	1 pkt.	160	7	½	2	14	3.0	20	450	0
French, reduced calorie	1 pkt.	160	23	1½	0	8	1.0	0	490	0
herb vinaigrette, fat free	1 pkt.	50	11	1	0	0	0.0	0	330	0
ranch	1 pkt.	230	10	½	1	21	3.0	20	550	0
Salads										
garden	1	35	7	½	2	0	0.0	0	20	3
grilled chicken deluxe	1	120	7	½	21	2	0.0	45	240	3
Sausage McMuffin®, w/ egg	1	440	27	2	19	28	10.0	255	890	1
Scrambled eggs	1 order	160	1	0	13	11	3.5	425	170	0
Shakes										
chocolate	small	360	60	4	11	9	6.0	40	250	1
strawberry	small	360	60	4	11	9	6.0	40	180	0
vanilla	small	360	59	4	11	9	6.0	40	250	0

FAST FOODS

McDonald's®

ITEM	AMOUNT	CALORIES	CARBOHYDRATE (g)	CARBOHYDRATE CHOICES	PROTEIN (g)	FAT (g)	SATURATED FAT (g)	CHOLESTEROL (mg)	SODIUM (mg)	FIBER (g)
Sundaes										
hot caramel	1	360	61	4	7	10	6.0	35	180	0
hot fudge	1	340	52	3½	8	12	9.0	30	170	1
strawberry	1	290	50	3	7	7	5.0	30	95	0
Value meals, regular,										
w/ medium drink & medium fries										
Big Mac®	1 meal	1220	160	10	32	53	14.0	85	1380	8
Chicken McNuggets®, 6 piece	1 meal	950	130	8	24	39	7.5	60	820	5
Crispy Chicken Deluxe™	1 meal	1160	158	10	32	47	8.0	55	1410	9
Filet-O-Fish®	1 meal	1100	157	10	22	47	8.5	50	1180	7
Quarter Pounder®	1 meal	1080	152	9½	29	43	12.0	70	1130	7
two cheeseburger	1 meal	1300	185	12	36	48	16.0	80	1950	9
Value meals, Super Size®,										
w/ large drink & Super Size® fries										
Big Mac®	1 meal	1410	199	12½	34	57	14.5	85	1450	9
Crispy Chicken Deluxe™	1 meal	1350	197	12½	34	51	9.5	55	1480	10
Filet-O-Fish®	1 meal	1300	196	12½	24	51	9.0	50	1250	8
Pizza Hut®										
Beef taco pizza										
hand tossed	1 slice	270	35	2	13	8	3.5	15	870	3
pan	1 slice	300	36	2½	12	12	4.5	15	770	3
Thin 'N Crispy®	1 slice	260	29	2	13	10	4.5	20	850	2
Breadstick	1	130	20	1	3	4	1.0	0	170	1
Buffalo wings										
hot	4	210	4	0	22	12	3.0	130	900	0
mild	5	200	0	0	23	12	3.5	150	510	0
Cheese pizza										
hand tossed	1 slice	309	43	3	14	9	5.0	11	848	3
pan	1 slice	361	44	3	13	15	5.5	11	678	3
Personal Pan Pizza®	1 pizza	813	110	7	31	27	12.0	24	1581	8
Sicilian	1 slice	295	32	2	12	13	6.5	11	815	3
stuffed crust	1 slice	445	46	3	22	19	10.0	24	1090	3
The Big New Yorker®	1 slice	393	42	3	20	17	8.5	19	1099	3
Thin 'N Crispy®	1 slice	243	27	2	11	10	5.0	11	653	2
Chicken supreme pizza										
hand tossed	1 slice	291	44	3	15	6	3.0	17	841	4
pan	1 slice	343	45	3	15	12	4.0	16	671	3
Sicilian	1 slice	269	32	2	13	10	5.0	15	732	3
stuffed crust	1 slice	432	47	3	24	17	8.0	32	1111	3
Thin 'N Crispy®	1 slice	232	29	2	13	7	3.0	19	681	3
Dessert pizza										
apple	1 slice	250	48	3	3	5	1.0	0	230	2

FAST FOODS

Pizza Hut®

ITEM	AMOUNT	CALORIES	CARBOHYDRATE (g)	CARBOHYDRATE CHOICES	PROTEIN (g)	FAT (g)	SATURATED FAT (g)	CHOLESTEROL (mg)	SODIUM (mg)	FIBER (g)
Dessert pizza *(con't.)*										
cherry	1 slice	250	47	3	3	5	1.0	0	220	3
Garlic bread	1 slice	150	16	1	3	8	1.5	0	240	1
Ham pizza										
hand tossed	1 slice	279	43	3	13	6	3.0	15	857	3
pan	1 slice	331	44	3	12	12	4.0	15	687	3
Sicilian	1 slice	257	30	2	11	10	5.0	14	745	3
stuffed crust	1 slice	404	45	3	24	22	12.5	39	1190	2
Thin 'N Crispy®	1 slice	212	27	2	10	7	3.0	15	662	2
Meat Lover's® pizza										
hand tossed	1 slice	376	44	3	17	15	6.5	30	1077	4
pan	1 slice	428	45	3	16	21	7.5	29	607	3
Sicilian	1 slice	344	31	2	14	18	8.0	27	948	3
stuffed crust	1 slice	543	46	3	26	29	12.5	48	1427	3
Thin 'N Crispy®	1 slice	339	28	2	15	19	8.0	35	970	3
Pasta										
Cavatini® pasta	1 order	480	66	4	21	14	6.0	8	1170	9
Cavatini Supreme® pasta	1 order	560	73	4	24	19	8.0	10	1400	10
spaghetti, w/ marinara	1 order	490	91	5½	18	6	1.0	0	730	8
spaghetti, w/ meat sauce	1 order	600	98	6	23	13	5.0	8	910	9
spaghetti, w/ meatballs	1 order	850	120	7	37	24	10.0	17	1120	10
Pepperoni Lover's® pizza										
hand tossed	1 slice	372	43	3	17	14	6.5	26	1123	3
pan	1 slice	370	44	3	13	16	5.5	18	767	3
Sicilian	1 slice	321	31	2	13	16	7.5	19	899	3
stuffed crust	1 slice	525	46	3	26	26	12.5	40	1413	3
Thin 'N Crispy®	1 slice	289	28	2	13	14	6.0	22	859	2
Pepperoni pizza										
hand tossed	1 slice	301	43	3	13	8	4.0	15	867	3
pan	1 slice	353	44	3	12	14	5.0	14	697	3
Personal Pan Pizza®	1 pizza	810	111	7	30	28	11.0	32	1661	8
Sicilian	1 slice	227	31	2	11	13	5.0	13	754	3
stuffed crust	1 slice	438	45	3	21	19	9.0	27	1116	2
The Big New Yorker®	1 slice	380	42	3	18	16	7.0	22	1116	3
Thin 'N Crispy®	1 slice	235	27	2	10	10	4.0	14	672	2
Sausage pizza										
hand tossed	1 slice	363	44	3	16	14	6.0	26	975	4
pan	1 slice	415	45	3	15	20	6.5	26	805	3
Sicilian	1 slice	333	31	2	13	18	7.5	24	855	3
stuffed crust	1 slice	478	46	3	22	23	10.5	35	1164	3
Thin 'N Crispy®	1 slice	325	28	2	14	18	7.0	32	865	3

FAST FOODS
Pizza Hut®

ITEM	AMOUNT	CALORIES	CARBOHYDRATE (g)	CARBOHYDRATE CHOICES	PROTEIN (g)	FAT (g)	SATURATED FAT (g)	CHOLESTEROL (mg)	SODIUM (mg)	FIBER (g)
Super supreme pizza										
hand tossed	1 slice	359	45	3	16	12	5.0	23	1024	4
pan	1 slice	401	46	3	15	18	6.0	22	854	4
Sicilian	1 slice	323	32	2	13	16	7.0	21	911	3
stuffed crust	1 slice	505	46	3	25	25	11.0	44	1371	3
Thin 'N Crispy®	1 slice	304	29	2	14	15	6.0	26	902	3
Supreme pizza										
hand tossed	1 slice	333	44	3	15	11	5.0	18	927	4
pan	1 slice	385	45	3	14	17	5.5	18	757	4
Personal Pan Pizza®	1 pizza	808	111	7	30	27	10.5	28	1579	8
Sicilian	1 slice	307	32	2	13	15	6.5	17	815	3
stuffed crust	1 slice	487	47	3	24	23	10.5	33	1227	3
The Big New Yorker®	1 slice	459	44	3	10	22	9.5	33	1310	4
Thin 'N Crispy®	1 slice	284	29	2	13	15	5.5	20	784	3
Supreme sandwich	1	640	62	4	34	28	10.0	28	2150	4
The Edge® pizza										
chicken veggie	1 slice	120	16	1	6	3	1.0	10	310	1
meaty	1 slice	150	15	1	7	7	3.0	15	430	1
taco	1 slice	140	17	1	6	6	2.0	10	450	1
the works	1 slice	140	16	1	6	5	2.0	10	390	1
veggie	1 slice	110	16	1	4	3	1.0	5	250	1
Veggie Lover's® pizza										
hand tossed	1 slice	281	45	3	12	6	3.0	7	771	4
pan	1 slice	333	46	3	11	12	4.0	7	601	4
Sicilian	1 slice	252	32	2	10	10	5.0	7	627	3
stuffed crust	1 slice	421	48	3	20	17	8.0	19	1039	3
Thin 'N Crispy®	1 slice	222	30	2	9	8	3.0	7	621	3
Subway®										
Bread										
deli style roll	1	170	31	2	6	2	1.0	0	350	1
wheat	1 (6 in.)	210	39	2½	8	3	1.0	0	430	3
white	1 (6 in.)	190	38	2½	7	1	1.0	0	420	0
Chicken breast sub	1 (6 in.)	342	46	3	26	6	2.0	48	966	3
Classic Italian B.M.T.®										
sub	1 (6 in.)	450	45	3	21	21	8.0	52	1579	3
super sub	1 (6 in.)	668	47	3	33	39	14.0	104	2576	3
Cold Cut Trio™										
sub	1 (6 in.)	374	45	3	19	14	5.0	47	1435	3
super sub	1 (6 in.)	517	47	3	29	24	8.0	93	2576	3
Condiments & extras										
bacon	2 strips	42	0	0	3	3	1.0	9	160	0
cheese, triangles	2	41	0	0	2	3	2.0	10	204	0

FAST FOODS
Subway®

ITEM	AMOUNT	CALORIES	CARBOHYDRATE (g)	CARBOHYDRATE CHOICES	PROTEIN (g)	FAT (g)	SATURATED FAT (g)	CHOLESTEROL (mg)	SODIUM (mg)	FIBER (g)
Condiments & extras *(con't.)*										
mayonnaise	1 tsp.	37	0	0	0	4	1.0	3	27	0
mayonnaise, light	1 tsp.	15	0	0	0	2	0.0	2	33	0
Cookies										
Brazil nut cookie	1	215	29	2	3	10	3.0	14	153	1
chocolate chip M&M®	1	212	29	2	2	10	3.0	13	144	1
chocolate chunk	1	215	29	2	2	10	3.0	13	144	1
macadamia nut cookie	1	222	28	2	2	11	2.0	12	144	1
oatmeal raisin	1	199	29	2	3	8	2.0	14	159	1
oatmeal raisin, lowfat	1	168	29	2	3	3	1.0	15	171	2
peanut butter	1	223	27	2	3	12	2.0	0	214	1
sugar	1	225	28	2	2	12	3.0	18	180	0
Ham										
deli style sandwich	1	224	37	2½	12	3	0.0	12	827	1
sub	1 (6 in.)	293	45	3	18	5	2.0	25	1342	3
Meatball										
sub	1 (6 in.)	413	50	3	19	15	6.0	35	1025	5
super sub	1 (6 in.)	594	58	3½	30	27	11.0	70	1468	7
Roast beef										
deli style sandwich	1	236	37	2½	14	4	0.0	13	678	1
sub	1 (6 in.)	296	45	3	19	5	2.0	20	928	3
Salad dressings										
Italian, creamy	1 T.	65	3	0	0	7	1.0	4	133	0
Italian, fat free	1 T.	5	1	0	0	0	0.0	0	153	0
ranch	1 T.	88	2	0	0	10	2.0	6	118	0
ranch, fat free	1 T.	15	4	0	0	0	0.0	0	178	0
Salads, w/o dressing										
chicken breast	1	162	13	1	20	4	1.0	48	693	1
Classic Italian B.M.T.®	1	269	11	1	14	19	7.0	52	1305	1
Cold Cut Trio™	1	193	12	1	12	12	4.0	47	1162	1
roast beef	1	115	11	1	12	3	1.0	20	654	1
Subway Club®	1	123	12	1	14	3	1.0	26	965	1
Subway Seafood & Crab®	1	157	17	1	7	7	1.0	14	761	2
tuna	1	198	11	1	11	12	2.0	32	669	1
turkey breast & ham	1	107	11	1	11	2	1.0	23	982	1
Veggie Delite®	1	51	10	½	2	1	0.0	0	308	1
Steak & cheese sub	1 (6 in.)	363	47	3	24	10	4.0	37	1160	4
Subway Club® sub	1 (6 in.)	304	46	3	21	5	2.0	26	1239	3
Subway Melt™ sub	1 (6 in.)	370	46	3	23	11	5.0	41	1619	3
Subway Seafood & Crab® sub	1 (6 in.)	338	51	3½	14	9	2.0	14	1034	3
Tuna										
deli style sandwich	1	267	37	2½	12	8	1.0	16	627	1

FAST FOODS
Subway®

ITEM	AMOUNT	CALORIES	CARBOHYDRATE (g)	CARBOHYDRATE CHOICES	PROTEIN (g)	FAT (g)	SATURATED FAT (g)	CHOLESTEROL (mg)	SODIUM (mg)	FIBER (g)
Tuna *(con't.)*										
sub	1 (6 in.)	378	45	3	18	14	3.0	32	942	3
Turkey breast										
deli style sandwich	1	227	37	2½	13	3	0.0	13	839	1
sub	1 (6 in.)	282	45	3	17	4	1.0	20	1170	3
super sub	1 (6 in.)	333	47	3	26	4	2.0	40	1758	3
Turkey breast & ham										
sub	1 (6 in.)	288	45	3	18	4	2.0	23	1256	3
super sub	1 (6 in.)	296	47	3	27	6	2.0	45	1929	3
Veggie Delite® sub	1 (6 in.)	232	43	3	9	3	1.0	0	582	3
Wraps										
chicken Parmesan ranch	1	333	56	4	17	5	2.0	45	1393	2
steak & cheese	1	353	53	3½	16	9	4.0	37	1450	2
turkey breast & bacon	1	355	52	3½	14	10	4.0	39	1823	1

Note: Subs & sandwiches do not
include cheese or mayonnaise.

Taco Bell®

ITEM	AMOUNT	CALORIES	CARBOHYDRATE (g)	CARBOHYDRATE CHOICES	PROTEIN (g)	FAT (g)	SATURATED FAT (g)	CHOLESTEROL (mg)	SODIUM (mg)	FIBER (g)
Big Beef MexiMelt®	1	290	23	1½	16	15	7.0	45	850	4
Burritos										
7-Layer	1	530	66	3½	16	23	7.0	25	1280	13
bacon cheeseburger	1	570	46	2½	27	31	12.0	70	1460	6
bean	1	380	55	3½	13	12	4.0	10	1100	13
Big Beef Supreme®	1	520	54	3	24	23	10.0	55	1520	11
Big Chicken Supreme®	1	510	52	3½	23	24	7.0	95	1900	4
Burrito Supreme®	1	440	51	3	17	19	8.0	35	1230	10
chicken club	1	540	43	3	20	32	10.0	80	1250	4
chili cheese	1	330	37	2	14	13	6.0	35	870	5
country breakfast	1	270	26	2	8	14	5.0	195	690	2
double bacon & egg	1	480	39	2½	18	27	9.0	400	1240	2
fiesta breakfast	1	280	25	1½	9	16	6.0	25	580	2
grande breakfast	1	420	43	3	13	22	7.0	205	1050	3
grilled chicken	1	410	50	3	17	15	4.5	55	1380	4
Choco Taco® ice cream	1	310	37	2½	3	17	10.0	20	100	1
Cinnamon twists	1 order	140	19	1	1	6	0.0	0	190	0
Gorditas, fiesta										
beef	1	290	31	2	14	13	4.0	25	880	3
grilled chicken	1	260	28	2	16	10	2.5	30	580	3
grilled steak	1	270	27	2	17	10	3.0	25	600	3
Gorditas, Santa Fe										
beef	1	380	33	2	14	20	4.0	35	440	4
grilled chicken	1	370	30	2	17	20	4.0	40	610	3

FAST FOODS
Taco Bell®

ITEM	AMOUNT	CALORIES	CARBOHYDRATE (g)	CARBOHYDRATE CHOICES	PROTEIN (g)	FAT (g)	SATURATED FAT (g)	CHOLESTEROL (mg)	SODIUM (mg)	FIBER (g)
Gorditas, Santa Fe *(con't.)*										
grilled steak	1	370	29	2	18	21	4.5	35	360	3
Gorditas, Supreme®										
beef	1	300	31	2	14	13	6.0	35	390	3
grilled chicken	1	300	28	2	17	14	5.0	45	540	3
grilled steak	1	310	27	2	17	14	5.0	35	550	3
Guacamole	¾ oz.	35	1	0	0	3	0.0	0	80	1
Hash brown nuggets	1 order	280	29	2	2	18	5.0	0	570	1
Mexican pizza	1	570	42	2	21	35	10.0	45	1040	8
Mexican rice	1 order	190	23	1½	5	9	3.5	15	760	1
Nachos										
Big Beef Supreme®	1 order	450	45	2½	14	24	8.0	30	810	9
Nachos BellGrande®	1 order	770	84	4½	21	39	11.0	35	1310	17
regular	1 order	320	34	2	5	18	4.0	5	570	3
Pintos 'n cheese	1 order	190	18	½	9	9	4.0	15	650	10
Quesadillas										
breakfast, w/ bacon	1	450	33	2	19	27	11.0	290	1200	2
breakfast, w/ cheese	1	380	33	2	15	21	9.0	280	1010	1
breakfast, w/ sausage	1	430	33	2	17	25	10.0	285	1090	1
cheese	1	350	32	2	16	18	9.0	50	860	2
chicken	1	410	34	2	23	21	10.0	90	1170	3
Taco salad, w/ salsa										
w/ shell	1	850	65	3	30	52	15.0	60	1780	16
w/o shell	1	420	32	1	24	22	11.0	60	1520	15
Tacos										
BLT soft	1	340	22	1½	11	23	8.0	40	610	2
Double Decker®	1	340	38	2	14	15	5.0	25	750	9
grilled chicken soft	1	240	21	1½	12	12	3.5	45	1110	3
grilled steak soft	1	230	20	1	15	10	2.5	25	1020	2
hard	1	180	12	1	9	10	4.0	25	330	3
soft	1	220	21	1½	11	10	4.5	25	580	3
Soft Taco Supreme®	1	260	23	1½	12	14	7.0	35	590	3
Taco Supreme®	1	220	14	1	10	14	7.0	35	350	3
Tostadas	1	300	31	1	10	15	5.0	15	650	12
Wendy's®										
Baked potatoes										
bacon & cheese	1	530	78	5	17	18	4.0	20	1390	7
broccoli & cheese	1	470	80	5	9	14	2.5	5	470	9
cheese	1	570	78	5	14	23	8.0	30	640	7
chili & cheese	1	630	83	5	20	24	9.0	40	770	9
plain	1	310	71	4	7	0	0.0	0	25	7
sour cream & chives	1	380	74	4½	8	6	4.0	15	40	8

FAST FOODS
Wendy's®

ITEM	AMOUNT	CALORIES	CARBOHYDRATE (g)	CARBOHYDRATE CHOICES	PROTEIN (g)	FAT (g)	SATURATED FAT (g)	CHOLESTEROL (mg)	SODIUM (mg)	FIBER (g)
Breadsticks, soft	1	130	23	1½	4	3	0.5	5	250	1
Chicken nuggets	5	230	11	1	11	16	3.0	30	470	0
Chicken sandwiches										
breaded chicken	1	440	44	3	28	18	3.5	60	840	2
chicken club	1	470	44	3	31	20	4.0	70	970	2
grilled chicken	1	310	35	2	27	8	1.5	65	790	2
Spicy Chicken™	1	410	43	3	28	15	2.5	65	1280	2
Chili	small	210	21	1	15	7	2.5	30	800	5
Chocolate chip cookies	1	270	36	2½	3	13	6.0	30	120	1
French fries										
small	1 order	270	35	2	4	13	2.0	0	85	3
biggie	1 order	470	61	3½	7	23	3.5	0	150	6
great biggie	1 order	570	73	4½	8	27	4.0	0	180	7
Fresh Stuffed Pitas®, w/ dressing										
chicken Caesar	1	490	48	3	34	18	5.0	65	1320	4
classic Greek	1	440	50	3	15	20	8.0	35	1050	4
garden ranch chicken	1	480	51	3	30	18	4.0	70	1180	5
garden veggie	1	400	52	3	11	17	3.5	20	760	5
Frosty dairy dessert										
small	1	330	56	4	8	8	5.0	35	200	0
medium	1	440	73	5	11	11	7.0	50	260	0
Hamburgers										
Big Bacon Classic®	1	580	46	3	34	30	12.0	100	1460	3
Classic Single™, plain	1	360	31	2	24	16	6.0	65	580	2
Classic Single™, w/ works	1	420	37	2½	25	20	7.0	70	920	3
Jr. bacon cheeseburger	1	380	34	2	20	19	7.0	60	850	2
Jr. cheeseburger	1	320	34	2	17	13	6.0	45	830	2
Jr. cheeseburger deluxe	1	360	36	2½	18	17	6.0	50	890	3
Jr. hamburger	1	270	34	2	15	10	3.5	30	610	2
Salad dressings										
French	2 T.	120	6	½	0	10	1.5	0	330	0
French, fat free	2 T.	35	8	½	0	0	0.0	0	150	0
Hidden Valley Ranch®	2 T.	100	1	0	1	10	1.5	10	220	0
Italian Caesar	2 T.	150	1	0	1	16	2.5	20	240	0
thousand island	2 T.	90	2	0	0	8	1.5	10	125	0
Salads, w/o dressing										
Caesar side	1	110	7	½	10	5	2.5	15	650	1
deluxe garden	1	110	9	½	7	6	1.0	0	350	3
grilled chicken	1	200	9	½	25	8	1.5	50	720	3
side	1	60	5	0	4	3	0.0	0	180	2
taco, w/ chips	1	530	50	3	27	26	10.0	60	1090	9

FATS, OILS, CREAM & GRAVY

ITEM	AMOUNT	CALORIES	CARBOHYDRATE (g)	CARBOHYDRATE CHOICES	PROTEIN (g)	FAT (g)	SATURATED FAT (g)	CHOLESTEROL (mg)	SODIUM (mg)	FIBER (g)
FATS, OILS, CREAM & GRAVY										
Bacon fat	1 T.	125	0	0	0	14	6.0	14	76	0
Beef fat/tallow	1 T.	116	0	0	0	13	6.5	14	0	0
Benecol® spread										
light	1 tsp.	20	0	0	0	2	0.0	0	43	0
regular	1 tsp.	30	0	0	0	3	0.5	0	43	0
Butter										
butter oil	1 T.	112	0	0	0	13	8.0	33	0	0
stick	1 tsp.	34	0	0	0	4	2.0	10	39	0
stick	1 T.	102	0	0	0	12	7.0	31	117	0
stick, unsalted	1 tsp.	34	0	0	0	4	3.0	10	0	0
whipped	1 tsp.	23	0	0	0	3	2.0	7	26	0
Butter flavored sprinkles	1 tsp.	5	2	0	0	0	0.0	0	120	0
Buttery spray	⅓ second	0	0	0	0	0	0.0	0	0	0
Chicken fat	1 T.	115	0	0	0	13	4.0	11	0	0
Coffee-Mate®										
fat free	1 T.	10	2	0	0	0	0.0	0	0	0
regular	1 T.	20	2	0	0	1	0.0	0	0	0
Coffee Rich®										
fat free	1 T.	15	2	0	0	0	0.0	0	10	0
regular	1 T.	20	2	0	0	2	0.0	0	10	0
Cooking spray	2 seconds	8	0	0	0	1	0.0	0	0	0
Cream										
heavy	1 T.	51	0	0	0	6	3.5	20	6	0
medium, 25% fat	1 T.	36	1	0	0	4	2.0	13	6	0
Gravy, beef										
au jus, can	¼ cup	10	1	0	1	0	0.0	0	30	0
brown, mix	¼ cup	19	3	0	1	0	0.0	0	269	0
fat free, can	¼ cup	20	5	0	0	0	0.0	0	310	0
homemade	¼ cup	45	3	0	2	3	1.0	2	384	0
mix	¼ cup	30	3	0	1	1	0.0	0	290	0
regular, can	¼ cup	31	3	0	2	1	0.5	2	326	0
Gravy, chicken										
fat free, can	¼ cup	15	3	0	0	0	0.0	0	320	0
giblet, hmde.	¼ cup	49	3	0	3	3	1.0	28	341	0
mix	¼ cup	21	4	0	1	0	0.0	1	283	0
regular, can	¼ cup	47	3	0	1	3	1.0	1	343	0
Gravy, other										
mushroom, can	¼ cup	30	3	0	1	2	0.0	0	339	0
onion, mix	¼ cup	20	4	0	1	0	0.0	0	253	0
pork, jar	¼ cup	25	3	0	1	1	0.0	0	340	0
sausage, can	¼ cup	70	5	0	2	5	1.5	5	300	0

FATS, OILS, CREAM & GRAVY

ITEM	AMOUNT	CALORIES	CARBOHYDRATE (g)	CARBOHYDRATE CHOICES	PROTEIN (g)	FAT (g)	SATURATED FAT (g)	CHOLESTEROL (mg)	SODIUM (mg)	FIBER (g)
Gravy, other *(con't.)*										
turkey, can	¼ cup	30	3	0	2	1	0.5	1	343	0
turkey, mix	¼ cup	22	4	0	1	0	0.0	1	374	0
vegetarian, brown, mix	¼ cup	15	3	0	0	0	0.0	0	270	0
Half & half										
fat free	1 T.	10	2	0	0	0	0.0	0	15	0
regular	1 T.	20	1	0	0	2	1.0	6	6	0
Lard/pork fat	1 T.	116	0	0	0	13	5.0	12	0	0
Margarine										
fat free	1 tsp.	34	0	0	0	4	1.0	0	35	0
light	1 tsp.	22	0	0	0	3	0.0	0	23	0
soft/tub	1 tsp.	34	0	0	0	4	1.0	0	51	0
soft/tub, unsalted	1 tsp.	34	0	0	0	4	1.0	0	0	0
stick	1 tsp.	34	0	0	0	4	0.5	0	44	0
stick	1 T.	101	0	0	0	11	2.0	0	133	0
Mayonnaise										
fat free	1 T.	10	2	0	0	0	0.0	0	105	0
imitation, soy	1 T.	35	1	0	0	3	0.0	0	105	0
lowfat	1 T.	36	3	0	0	3	1.0	4	78	0
regular	1 T.	100	0	0	0	11	2.0	10	75	0
Miracle Whip®										
Free®	1 T.	15	2	0	0	0	0.0	0	125	0
light	1 T.	36	3	0	0	3	0.0	4	99	0
regular	1 T.	57	4	0	0	5	1.0	4	104	0
Mocha Mix®										
fat free	1 T.	10	1	0	0	0	0.0	0	5	0
regular	1 T.	20	1	0	0	2	0.0	0	5	0
Oils										
avocado	1 T.	124	0	0	0	14	1.5	0	0	0
canola	1 T.	120	0	0	0	14	1.0	0	0	0
chili	1 T.	130	0	0	0	14	2.0	0	0	0
coconut	1 T.	117	0	0	0	14	12.0	0	0	0
cod liver/fish	1 T.	123	0	0	0	14	3.0	78	0	0
corn	1 T.	120	0	0	0	14	2.0	0	0	0
cottonseed	1 T.	120	0	0	0	14	3.5	0	0	0
flaxseed/linseed	1 T.	120	0	0	0	14	1.5	0	0	0
grapeseed	1 T.	120	0	0	0	14	1.5	0	0	0
olive	1 T.	120	0	0	0	14	2.0	0	0	0
palm	1 T.	120	0	0	0	14	7.0	0	0	0
palm kernel	1 T.	117	0	0	0	14	11.0	0	0	0
peanut	1 T.	119	0	0	0	14	2.5	0	0	0
safflower	1 T.	120	0	0	0	14	1.0	0	0	0

FATS, OILS, CREAM & GRAVY

ITEM	AMOUNT	CALORIES	CARBOHYDRATE (g)	CARBOHYDRATE CHOICES	PROTEIN (g)	FAT (g)	SATURATED FAT (g)	CHOLESTEROL (mg)	SODIUM (mg)	FIBER (g)
Oils *(con't.)*										
sesame	1 T.	120	0	0	0	14	2.0	0	0	0
soybean	1 T.	120	0	0	0	14	2.0	0	0	0
sunflower	1 T.	120	0	0	0	14	1.5	0	0	0
walnut	1 T.	120	0	0	0	14	1.0	0	0	0
wheat germ	1 T.	120	0	0	0	14	2.5	0	0	0
Popcorn topping	1 T.	120	0	0	0	14	2.0	0	0	0
Shortening, vegetable	1 T.	113	0	0	0	13	3.0	0	0	0
Sour cream										
fat free	1 T.	18	3	0	1	0	0.0	1	13	0
imitation, soy	1 T.	25	1	0	1	3	1.0	0	60	0
light	1 T.	20	1	0	1	1	1.0	5	10	0
regular	1 T.	31	1	0	0	3	2.0	6	8	0

FISH & SEAFOOD
Cooked w/o fat unless indicated

ITEM	AMOUNT	CALORIES	CARBOHYDRATE (g)	CARBOHYDRATE CHOICES	PROTEIN (g)	FAT (g)	SATURATED FAT (g)	CHOLESTEROL (mg)	SODIUM (mg)	FIBER (g)
Abalone, breaded & fried	3 oz.	161	9	½	17	6	1.5	80	503	0
Anchovies, oil pack, can	3	25	0	0	3	1	0.0	10	440	0
Anchovy paste	1 tsp.	14	0	0	1	1	0.0	4	874	0
Bass										
freshwater	3 oz.	124	0	0	21	4	1.0	74	77	0
sea/striped	3 oz.	105	0	0	20	2	0.5	45	74	0
Bluefish	3 oz.	135	0	0	22	5	1.0	65	65	0
Burbot	3 oz.	98	0	0	21	1	0.0	65	105	0
Butterfish	3 oz.	159	0	0	19	9	2.5	71	97	0
Calamari/squid										
baked/broiled	1 cup	193	5	0	26	7	1.5	393	518	0
breaded & fried	1 cup	263	12	1	27	11	3.0	390	459	0
Carp										
baked/broiled	3 oz.	138	0	0	19	6	1.5	71	54	0
breaded & fried	3 oz.	236	10	½	18	13	3.0	85	441	1
Catfish, farmed										
baked/broiled	3 oz.	129	0	0	16	7	1.5	54	68	0
breaded & fried	3 oz.	244	10	½	16	15	3.5	69	450	1
Catfish, wild	3 oz.	89	0	0	16	2	0.5	61	43	0
Caviar, black/red	1 T.	40	1	0	4	3	1.0	94	240	0
Cisco, smoked	3 oz.	151	0	0	14	10	1.5	27	409	0
Clams										
breaded & fried	9 small	172	9	½	12	10	2.0	52	310	0
raw	6 large	89	3	1	15	1	0.0	41	67	0
stuffed, frzn.	1 (2.5 oz.)	130	15	1	6	6	0.5	0	530	2

FISH & SEAFOOD

ITEM	AMOUNT	CALORIES	CARBOHYDRATE (g)	CARBOHYDRATE CHOICES	PROTEIN (g)	FAT (g)	SATURATED FAT (g)	CHOLESTEROL (mg)	SODIUM (mg)	FIBER (g)
Cod, Atlantic/Pacific										
baked/broiled	3 oz.	89	0	0	19	1	0.0	47	66	0
breaded & fried	3 oz.	147	6	½	15	7	2.0	48	93	0
dried, salted	3 oz.	247	0	0	53	2	0.5	129	5976	0
Crab										
Alaska King	3 oz.	83	0	0	17	1	0.0	45	911	0
blue, can	½ cup	67	0	0	14	1	0.0	60	225	0
blue, fresh	3 oz.	87	0	0	17	2	0.0	85	237	0
dungeness	3 oz.	94	1	0	19	1	0.0	65	321	0
imitation	3 oz.	87	9	½	10	1	0.0	17	715	0
snow	3 oz.	117	0	0	16	5	1.0	80	459	0
soft shell, breaded & fried	3 oz.	284	15	1	17	17	4.0	104	439	1
Crab cakes	1 (2 oz.)	160	5	0	11	10	2.0	82	491	0
Crawdads/crayfish	3 oz.	75	0	0	14	1	0.0	113	80	0
Croaker, breaded & fried	3 oz.	188	6	½	15	11	3.0	71	296	0
Cusk	3 oz.	95	0	0	21	1	0.0	45	34	0
Cuttlefish	3 oz.	134	1	0	28	1	0.0	191	633	0
Dolphinfish/mahi mahi	3 oz.	93	0	0	20	1	0.0	80	96	0
Drum, freshwater	3 oz.	130	0	0	19	5	1.0	70	82	0
Eel	3 oz.	201	0	0	20	13	3.5	137	55	0
Escargot/snails	6	54	1	0	10	1	0.0	30	36	0
Fish cakes, breaded, frzn.	1 (3 oz.)	230	15	1	8	15	6.0	22	150	1
Fish fillets, frzn.	1 (3.7 oz.)	130	0	0	18	6	1.0	60	230	0
Fish sticks, frzn.	4	310	27	2	18	14	4.0	128	663	1
Flounder										
baked/broiled	3 oz.	100	0	0	21	1	0.0	58	89	0
breaded & fried	3 oz.	185	7	½	17	10	2.5	58	329	0
Gefiltefish	3 oz.	71	6	½	8	1	0.0	26	446	0
Grouper	3 oz.	100	0	0	21	1	0.5	40	45	0
Haddock										
baked/broiled	3 oz.	95	0	0	21	1	0.0	63	74	0
breaded & fried	3 oz.	199	11	1	16	10	2.0	72	393	1
smoked	3 oz.	99	0	0	21	1	0.0	65	649	0
Halibut										
Atlantic/Pacific	3 oz.	119	0	0	23	3	0.5	35	59	0
Greenland	3 oz.	203	0	0	16	15	4.0	50	88	0
Herring										
Atlantic, baked/broiled	3 oz.	173	0	0	20	10	2.0	65	98	0
Atlantic, pickled	1 (0.5 oz.)	39	1	0	2	3	0.0	2	131	0
Pacific, baked broiled	3 oz.	213	0	0	18	15	3.0	84	81	0
Ling/lingcod	3 oz.	94	0	0	21	1	0.0	43	147	0

FISH & SEAFOOD

ITEM	AMOUNT	CALORIES	CARBOHYDRATE (g)	CARBOHYDRATE CHOICES	PROTEIN (g)	FAT (g)	SATURATED FAT (g)	CHOLESTEROL (mg)	SODIUM (mg)	FIBER (g)
Lobster										
Northern, breaded & fried	3 oz.	180	7	½	16	9	2.5	68	327	0
Northern, broiled/steamed	3 oz.	99	1	0	17	3	1.5	65	529	0
spiny, steamed	3 oz.	122	3	0	22	2	0.5	77	193	0
Lox/smoked salmon	3 oz.	100	0	0	16	4	1.0	20	1701	0
Mackerel										
Atlantic	3 oz.	223	0	0	20	15	4.0	64	71	0
Jack/Pacific	3 oz.	171	0	0	22	9	2.0	51	94	0
king	3 oz.	114	0	0	22	2	0.5	58	173	0
Spanish	3 oz.	134	0	0	20	5	1.5	62	56	0
Milkfish	3 oz.	162	0	0	22	7	2.0	57	78	0
Mollusks/whelk	3 oz.	234	13	1	41	1	0.0	111	350	0
Monkfish	3 oz.	83	0	0	16	2	0.5	27	20	0
Mullet, striped	3 oz.	128	0	0	21	4	1.0	54	60	0
Mussels	3 oz.	146	6	½	20	4	1.0	48	314	0
Octopus	3 oz.	139	4	0	25	2	0.5	82	391	0
Orange roughy	3 oz.	76	0	0	16	1	0.0	22	69	0
Oysters										
Eastern, breaded & fried	6	174	10	½	8	11	3.5	71	368	0
Eastern, raw	6	58	3	0	6	2	0.5	46	94	0
Pacific, raw	6	69	4	0	8	2	0.5	43	90	0
smoked, oil pack, can	6	190	9	½	14	11	3.0	55	340	0
Perch										
baked/broiled	3 oz.	103	0	0	20	2	0.5	46	82	0
breaded & fried	3 oz.	187	7	½	17	10	2.5	54	324	0
Pollock, Atlantic	3 oz.	100	0	0	21	1	0.0	77	94	0
Pompano	3 oz.	179	0	0	20	11	4.0	54	65	0
Pout	3 oz.	87	0	0	18	1	0.5	57	66	0
Rockfish, Pacific	3 oz.	103	0	0	20	2	0.5	37	65	0
Roe	3 oz.	174	2	0	24	7	1.5	407	100	0
Sablefish	3 oz.	213	0	0	15	17	3.5	54	61	0
Salmon										
Atlantic	3 oz.	155	0	0	22	7	1.0	60	48	0
Chinook	3 oz.	197	0	0	22	11	2.5	72	51	0
coho	3 oz.	151	0	0	21	7	1.5	54	44	0
pink, can	3 oz.	122	0	0	16	7	1.5	54	365	0
sockeye, can	3 oz.	130	0	0	17	6	1.5	37	458	0
Sardines, oil pack, can	2	50	0	0	6	3	0.0	34	121	0
Scallops										
bay, baked/broiled	3 oz.	122	2	0	22	1	0.0	56	263	0
imitation	3 oz.	84	9	½	11	0	0.0	19	676	0
sea, baked/broiled	6 large	120	2	0	22	1	0.0	55	260	0

FISH & SEAFOOD

ITEM	AMOUNT	CALORIES	CARBOHYDRATE (g)	CARBOHYDRATE CHOICES	PROTEIN (g)	FAT (g)	SATURATED FAT (g)	CHOLESTEROL (mg)	SODIUM (mg)	FIBER (g)
Scallops *(con't.)*										
sea, breaded & fried	6 large	200	9	½	17	10	2.5	57	432	0
Scup	3 oz.	115	0	0	21	3	1.0	57	46	0
Shad	3 oz.	214	0	0	18	15	4.0	82	55	0
Shad roe	½ cup	182	2	0	24	10	2.0	397	471	0
Shark	3 oz.	152	0	0	21	7	1.5	51	341	0
Shrimp										
baked/broiled/raw	10 large	54	0	0	12	1	0.0	107	123	0
breaded & fried	10 large	182	9	½	16	9	1.5	133	258	0
Smelt, rainbow										
baked/broiled	3 oz.	105	0	0	19	3	0.5	77	65	0
breaded & fried	3 oz.	212	10	½	17	11	2.5	88	456	1
Snapper	3 oz.	109	0	0	22	1	0.0	40	48	0
Sole										
baked/broiled	3 oz.	100	0	0	21	1	0.0	58	89	0
breaded & fried	3 oz.	185	7	½	17	10	2.5	58	329	0
Sturgeon										
baked/broiled	3 oz.	196	7	½	15	12	3.0	68	307	1
smoked	3 oz.	147	0	0	27	4	1.0	68	629	0
Sucker, white	3 oz.	101	0	0	18	3	0.5	45	43	0
Sunfish	3 oz.	97	0	0	21	1	0.0	73	88	0
Sushi, w/ rice & vegetables	½ cup	119	24	1½	4	0	0.0	6	172	1
Swordfish	3 oz.	132	0	0	22	4	1.0	43	98	0
Tilefish	3 oz.	125	0	0	21	4	0.5	54	50	0
Trout, rainbow										
baked/broiled	3 oz.	128	0	0	19	5	1.0	59	48	0
breaded & fried	3 oz.	227	8	½	20	12	2.5	72	360	0
Tuna, can										
light, oil pack	¼ cup	110	0	0	13	6	1.0	30	250	0
light, water pack	¼ cup	60	0	0	13	1	0.0	30	250	0
low sodium, water pack	¼ cup	70	0	0	15	1	0.0	25	35	0
white, oil pack	¼ cup	90	0	0	14	3	0.5	25	250	0
white, water pack	¼ cup	70	0	0	15	1	0.0	25	250	0
Tuna, fresh										
bluefin	3 oz.	156	0	0	25	5	1.5	42	43	0
yellowfin	3 oz.	118	0	0	26	1	0.5	49	40	0
Turbot	3 oz.	104	0	0	18	3	0.5	53	163	0
Walleye	3 oz.	101	0	0	21	1	0.5	94	55	0
Whitefish	3 oz.	146	0	0	21	6	1.0	65	55	0
Whiting	3 oz.	99	0	0	20	1	0.5	71	112	0
Wolffish, Atlantic	3 oz.	105	0	0	19	3	0.5	50	93	0
Yellowtail	3 oz.	159	0	0	25	6	1.0	60	43	0

FRUIT & VEGETABLE JUICES

ITEM	AMOUNT	CALORIES	CARBOHYDRATE (g)	CARBOHYDRATE CHOICES	PROTEIN (g)	FAT (g)	SATURATED FAT (g)	CHOLESTEROL (mg)	SODIUM (mg)	FIBER (g)
FRUIT & VEGETABLE JUICES										
Fruit Juices & Nectars										
Apple cider/juice	1 cup	117	29	2	0	0	0.0	0	7	0
Apple-cherry	1 cup	117	29	2	1	0	0.0	0	6	1
Apricot nectar	1 cup	141	36	2½	1	0	0.0	0	8	2
Cranberry cocktail										
reduced calorie	1 cup	45	11	1	0	0	0.0	0	7	0
regular	1 cup	144	36	2½	0	0	0.0	0	5	0
Five Alive®	1 cup	110	30	2	0	0	0.0	0	0	0
Grape										
purple, sweetened	1 cup	150	37	2½	0	0	0.0	0	0	0
purple, unsweetened	1 cup	160	41	3	0	0	0.0	0	0	0
white, unsweetened	1 cup	140	35	2	0	0	0.0	0	40	0
Grapefruit	1 cup	96	23	1½	1	0	0.0	0	2	0
Guava nectar	1 cup	149	38	2½	0	0	0.0	0	7	2
Kiwi-strawberry	1 cup	120	31	2	0	0	0.0	0	10	0
Lemon	2 T.	8	3	0	0	0	0.0	0	0	0
Lime	2 T.	8	3	0	0	0	0.0	0	0	0
Mango	1 cup	130	33	2	0	0	0.0	0	35	0
Orange	1 cup	110	25	1½	2	0	0.0	0	2	1
Passion fruit	1 cup	126	34	2	1	0	0.0	0	15	0
Peach juice/nectar	1 cup	134	35	2	1	0	0.0	0	17	1
Pear juice/nectar	1 cup	150	40	2½	0	0	0.0	0	10	2
Pineapple, unsweetened	1 cup	140	35	2	1	0	0.0	0	3	0
Prune	1 cup	182	45	3	2	0	0.0	0	10	3
Tropicana Twister®	1 cup	130	34	2	0	0	0.0	0	30	0
Vegetable Juices										
Beefamato®	1 cup	50	11	1	0	0	0.0	0	830	0
Carrot	1 cup	94	22	1½	2	0	0.0	0	68	2
Clamato®	1 cup	60	11	1	1	0	0.0	0	880	1
Tomato	1 cup	50	9	½	2	0	0.0	0	860	1
V-8®										
Healthy Request™	1 cup	50	12	1	1	0	0.0	0	460	1
regular	1 cup	50	10	½	1	0	0.0	0	620	1
regular, low sodium	1 cup	60	11	1	2	0	0.0	0	140	2
Splash®, tropical blend	1 cup	120	30	2	0	0	0.0	0	20	0
FRUITS										
Apples										
dried	4 rings	62	17	1	0	0	0.0	0	22	2

FRUITS

ITEM	AMOUNT	CALORIES	CARBOHYDRATE (g)	CARBOHYDRATE CHOICES	PROTEIN (g)	FAT (g)	SATURATED FAT (g)	CHOLESTEROL (mg)	SODIUM (mg)	FIBER (g)
Apples *(con't.)*										
fresh	1 medium	81	21	1½	0	1	0.0	0	0	4
Applesauce										
natural/unsweetened	½ cup	52	14	1	0	0	0.0	0	2	1
sweetened	½ cup	97	25	1½	0	0	0.0	0	4	1
Apricots										
dried	4 halves	42	11	1	1	0	0.0	0	1	2
fresh	1 medium	17	4	0	0	0	0.0	0	0	1
heavy syrup, can	½ cup	107	28	2	1	0	0.0	0	5	2
light syrup, can	½ cup	80	21	1½	1	0	0.0	0	5	1
Avocados	½ medium	162	7	0	2	15	2.5	0	10	5
Banana chips	½ cup	239	27	2	1	15	13.0	0	3	4
Bananas, fresh	1 medium	109	28	2	1	1	0.0	0	1	3
Blackberries, fresh	1 cup	75	18	½	1	1	0.0	0	0	8
Blueberries, fresh/frzn.	1 cup	81	20	1	1	1	0.0	0	9	4
Boysenberries, fresh	1 cup	75	18	½	1	1	0.0	0	0	8
Breadfruit, fresh	¼ medium	99	26	1½	1	0	0.0	0	2	5
Cantaloupe, fresh	1 cup	56	13	1	1	0	0.0	0	14	1
Casaba melon, fresh	1 cup	44	11	1	2	0	0.0	0	20	1
Cherries, red										
maraschino	1 medium	10	2	0	0	0	0.0	0	0	0
sour, fresh	½ cup	39	9	½	1	0	0.0	0	2	1
sour, heavy syrup, can	½ cup	116	30	2	1	0	0.0	0	9	1
sweet, fresh	12 medium	59	14	1	1	1	0.0	0	0	2
sweet, heavy syrup, can	½ cup	105	27	2	1	0	0.0	0	4	2
Coconut, shredded										
fresh	¼ cup	71	3	0	1	7	6.0	0	4	2
sweetened, dried	¼ cup	116	11	1	1	8	7.0	0	61	1
Cranberries										
Craisins®/sweetened, dried	¼ cup	98	25	1½	0	0	0.0	0	1	2
fresh/frzn.	½ cup	23	6	½	0	0	0.0	0	0	2
Currants, fresh	½ cup	35	9	½	1	0	0.0	0	1	4
Dates, dried	¼ cup	122	33	2	1	0	0.0	0	1	3
Figs										
dried	2 medium	105	25	1	1	0	0.0	0	5	5
fresh	2 medium	74	19	1	1	0	0.0	0	1	3
Fruit cocktail										
heavy syrup, can	½ cup	91	23	1½	0	0	0.0	0	7	1
light syrup, can	½ cup	69	18	1	0	0	0.0	0	7	1
Gooseberries, fresh	1 cup	66	15	½	1	1	0.0	0	2	6
Grapefruit										
light syrup, can	½ cup	76	20	1	1	0	0.0	0	3	1

FRUITS

ITEM	AMOUNT	CALORIES	CARBOHYDRATE (g)	CARBOHYDRATE CHOICES	PROTEIN (g)	FAT (g)	SATURATED FAT (g)	CHOLESTEROL (mg)	SODIUM (mg)	FIBER (g)
Grapefruit *(con't.)*										
sections, fresh	1 cup	74	19	1	1	0	0.0	0	0	3
whole, fresh	½ medium	39	10	½	1	0	0.0	0	0	1
Grapes, fresh	17 medium	60	15	1	1	0	0.0	0	2	1
Guavas, fresh	1 medium	46	11	½	1	1	0.0	0	3	5
Honeydew melon, fresh	1 cup	60	16	1	1	0	0.0	0	17	1
Kiwifruit, fresh	1 medium	46	11	1	1	0	0.0	0	4	3
Kumquats, fresh	1 medium	12	3	0	0	0	0.0	0	1	1
Lemons, fresh	½ medium	8	3	0	0	0	0.0	0	1	1
Limes, fresh	½ medium	10	4	0	0	0	0.0	0	1	1
Loganberries, fresh	1 cup	75	18	½	1	1	0.0	0	0	8
Mandarin oranges, can	½ cup	47	12	1	1	0	0.0	0	6	1
Mangoes, fresh	½ medium	67	18	1	1	0	0.0	0	2	2
Melon balls, frzn.	1 cup	57	14	1	1	0	0.0	0	54	1
Mixed fruit										
dried	¼ cup	83	22	1½	1	0	0.0	0	6	3
sweetened, frzn.	1 cup	245	61	4	4	0	0.0	0	8	5
Mulberries, fresh	1 cup	60	14	1	2	1	0.0	0	14	2
Nectarines, fresh	1 medium	67	16	1	1	1	0.0	0	0	2
Oranges, fresh	1 medium	62	15	1	1	0	0.0	0	0	2
Papayas, fresh	½ medium	59	15	1	1	0	0.0	0	5	3
Passion fruit, fresh	1 medium	17	4	0	0	0	0.0	0	5	2
Peaches										
fresh	1 medium	42	11	1	1	0	0.0	0	0	2
heavy syrup, can	½ cup	97	26	2	1	0	0.0	0	8	2
light syrup, can	½ cup	68	18	1	1	0	0.0	0	6	2
Pears										
fresh	1 medium	98	25	1½	1	1	0.0	0	0	4
heavy syrup, can	½ cup	98	26	2	0	0	0.0	0	7	2
light syrup, can	½ cup	72	19	1	0	0	0.0	0	6	2
Persimmons, native, fresh	1 medium	32	8	½	0	0	0.0	0	0	0
Pineapple chunks										
fresh	1 cup	76	19	1	1	1	0.0	0	2	2
heavy syrup, can	½ cup	99	26	2	0	0	0.0	0	1	1
light syrup, can	½ cup	66	17	1	0	0	0.0	0	1	1
Plantains, cooked	1 cup	179	48	3	1	0	0.0	0	8	4
Plums, fresh	1 medium	36	9	½	1	0	0.0	0	0	1
Pomegranates, fresh	½ medium	52	13	1	1	0	0.0	0	2	0
Prickly pears, fresh	1 medium	42	10	½	1	1	0.0	0	5	4
Prunes, dried	3 medium	60	16	1	1	0	0.0	0	1	2
Quince, fresh	1 medium	52	14	1	0	0	0.0	0	4	2
Raisins	¼ cup	124	33	2	1	0	0.0	0	5	2

FRUITS

ITEM	AMOUNT	CALORIES	CARBOHYDRATE (g)	CARBOHYDRATE CHOICES	PROTEIN (g)	FAT (g)	SATURATED FAT (g)	CHOLESTEROL (mg)	SODIUM (mg)	FIBER (g)
Raspberries, fresh	1 cup	60	14	½	1	1	0.0	0	0	8
Rhubarb										
fresh	1 cup	26	6	½	1	0	0.0	0	5	2
sweetened, cooked	½ cup	139	37	2½	0	0	0.0	0	1	2
Starfruit, fresh	1 medium	42	10	½	1	0	0.0	0	3	3
Strawberries										
fresh	1 cup	50	12	1	1	1	0.0	0	2	4
sweetened, frzn.	1 cup	245	66	4	1	0	0.0	0	8	5
Tangerines, fresh	1 medium	37	9	½	1	0	0.0	0	1	2
Tropical fruit, light, can	½ cup	80	21	1½	0	0	0.0	0	10	1
Watermelon, fresh	1 cup	49	11	1	1	1	0.0	0	3	1

MEATS
Cooked w/o fat unless indicated
Beef

ITEM	AMOUNT	CALORIES	CARBOHYDRATE (g)	CARBOHYDRATE CHOICES	PROTEIN (g)	FAT (g)	SATURATED FAT (g)	CHOLESTEROL (mg)	SODIUM (mg)	FIBER (g)
Bottom round	3 oz.	187	0	0	27	8	3.0	82	43	0
Chuck roast										
arm	3 oz.	184	0	0	28	7	2.5	86	56	0
blade	3 oz.	213	0	0	26	11	4.0	90	60	0
Corned brisket	3 oz.	213	0	0	15	16	5.0	83	964	0
Eye of round	3 oz.	165	0	0	24	7	3.0	60	52	0
Filet mignon	3 oz.	179	0	0	24	9	3.0	71	54	0
Flank steak	3 oz.	176	0	0	23	9	4.0	57	71	0
Ground										
extra lean, 9%	3 oz.	191	0	0	23	10	4.0	41	82	0
lean, 16%	3 oz.	213	0	0	21	14	6.0	70	42	0
lean, 18%	3 oz.	238	0	0	24	15	6.0	86	76	0
regular, 21%	3 oz.	244	0	0	20	18	8.0	74	51	0
London broil	3 oz.	176	0	0	23	9	4.0	57	71	0
Porterhouse steak	3 oz.	185	0	0	24	9	4.0	68	56	0
Pot roast, round	3 oz.	234	0	0	24	14	6.5	82	43	0
Prime rib	3 oz.	354	0	0	17	31	13.0	74	52	0
Rib eye steak	3 oz.	191	0	0	24	10	4.0	68	59	0
Round steak	3 oz.	205	0	0	23	12	5.0	61	50	0
Rump roast	3 oz.	220	0	0	25	13	5.0	82	43	0
Short ribs	3 oz.	251	0	0	26	15	7.0	79	49	0
Sirloin steak	3 oz.	172	0	0	26	7	3.0	76	56	0
Sirloin tips	3 oz.	157	0	0	24	6	2.0	69	55	0
Stew meat	3 oz.	259	0	0	24	18	7.0	85	250	0
Strip steak	3 oz.	176	0	0	24	8	3.0	65	58	0
T-bone steak	3 oz.	182	0	0	24	9	4.0	68	56	0
Tenderloin, lean	3 oz.	179	0	0	24	9	4.0	71	54	0

MEATS
Beef

ITEM	AMOUNT	CALORIES	CARBOHYDRATE (g)	CARBOHYDRATE CHOICES	PROTEIN (g)	FAT (g)	SATURATED FAT (g)	CHOLESTEROL (mg)	SODIUM (mg)	FIBER (g)
Top round	3 oz.	153	0	0	27	4	1.5	71	52	0
Top sirloin	3 oz.	166	0	0	26	6	2.5	76	56	0
Veal										
chops, breaded & fried	3 oz.	194	8	½	23	8	2.5	95	386	0
cutlets/loin chop, braised	3 oz.	242	0	0	26	15	6.0	100	68	0
loin	3 oz.	149	0	0	22	6	2.0	90	82	0
patties, breaded & fried	3 oz.	224	7	½	18	14	5.0	86	333	0
shoulder	3 oz.	235	0	0	19	17	7.0	78	56	0
sirloin	3 oz.	142	0	0	22	5	2.0	88	72	0
Game										
Beefalo	3 oz.	160	0	0	26	5	2.0	49	70	0
Bison/buffalo	3 oz.	122	0	0	24	2	1.0	70	48	0
Rabbit										
domestic	3 oz.	168	0	0	25	7	2.0	70	40	0
wild	3 oz.	147	0	0	28	3	1.0	105	38	0
Venison	3 oz.	134	0	0	26	3	1.0	95	46	0
Lamb										
Chops	3 oz.	184	0	0	26	8	3.0	81	71	0
Leg	3 oz.	219	0	0	22	14	6.0	79	56	0
Shoulder	3 oz.	235	0	0	19	17	7.0	78	56	0
Pork										
Chops										
broiled	3 oz.	179	0	0	24	8	3.0	67	54	0
fried	3 oz.	219	0	0	25	13	4.5	66	47	0
Ground	3 oz.	253	0	0	22	18	6.5	80	62	0
Ham										
cured, lean	3 oz.	134	0	0	21	5	1.5	47	1129	0
hocks	3 oz.	278	0	0	24	20	7.0	92	271	0
leg, fresh	3 oz.	232	0	0	23	15	5.5	80	51	0
picnic/shoulder roast	3 oz.	194	0	0	23	11	3.5	81	68	0
Loin	3 oz.	206	0	0	23	12	4.5	68	53	0
Spareribs, lean	3 oz.	199	0	0	22	12	4.0	73	54	0
Tenderloin, lean	3 oz.	139	0	0	24	4	1.5	67	48	0
Processed & Luncheon Meats										
Bacon	1 slice	36	0	0	2	3	1.0	5	101	0
Bacon bits										
imitation	1 T.	20	1	0	2	1	0.0	0	80	0
real	1 T.	30	0	0	3	2	1.0	5	250	0
Beef jerky	1 oz.	90	3	0	12	1	0.5	26	580	1
Beef sticks	2 (3.5 in.)	84	1	0	4	8	3.5	10	228	0
Bologna										
beef/beef & pork	1 oz.	88	0	0	3	8	3.5	16	278	0

MEATS
Processed & Luncheon Meats

ITEM	AMOUNT	CALORIES	CARBOHYDRATE (g)	CARBOHYDRATE CHOICES	PROTEIN (g)	FAT (g)	SATURATED FAT (g)	CHOLESTEROL (mg)	SODIUM (mg)	FIBER (g)
Bologna *(con't.)*										
Healthy Choice®	1 oz.	40	3	0	3	2	0.5	15	240	0
Braunschweiger	1 oz.	102	1	0	4	9	3.0	44	324	0
Canadian bacon	1 oz.	45	0	0	6	2	1.0	14	399	0
Corned beef, can	2 oz.	130	0	0	15	7	3.0	50	580	0
Corned beef hash, can	1 cup	398	24	1½	19	25	12.0	73	1188	1
Deviled ham® spread	¼ cup	140	3	0	7	11	3.5	30	410	0
Ham, chopped, can	2 oz.	90	0	0	9	6	2.0	30	600	0
Ham, deli, extra-lean	1 oz.	37	0	0	6	1	0.5	13	405	0
Headcheese	1 oz.	60	0	0	5	4	1.5	23	356	0
Hot dogs										
beef/pork & turkey	1 (1.6 oz.)	143	1	0	5	13	6.0	29	458	0
Healthy Choice®	1 (1.4 oz.)	60	5	0	5	2	0.5	10	320	0
Liverwurst	1 oz.	92	1	0	4	8	3.0	45	244	0
Mortadella	1 oz.	88	1	0	5	7	2.5	16	353	0
Olive loaf	1 oz.	70	2	0	3	6	2.0	20	360	0
Pastrami	1 oz.	99	1	0	5	8	3.0	26	348	0
Pepperoni	1 oz.	141	1	0	6	12	5.0	22	578	0
Roast beef, deli	1 oz.	32	0	0	6	1	0.0	14	287	0
Salami										
beef	1 oz.	74	1	0	4	6	2.5	18	333	0
beef & pork/Genoa	1 oz.	111	0	0	6	10	3.0	29	518	0
Sandwich steaks, frzn.	1 (2 oz.)	190	0	0	9	17	7.0	35	55	0
Sausages										
bockwurst	1 (2 oz.)	174	0	0	8	16	6.0	33	627	0
bratwurst	1 (2 oz.)	256	2	0	12	22	8.0	51	473	0
breakfast	1 (0.5 oz.)	56	0	0	2	5	2.0	9	135	0
chorizo	1 (2 oz.)	273	1	0	15	23	8.5	53	741	0
Italian	1 (2 oz.)	216	1	0	13	17	6.0	52	618	0
kielbasa	1 (2 oz.)	176	1	0	8	15	6.0	38	610	0
knockwurst	1 (2 oz.)	175	1	0	7	16	6.0	33	573	0
Polish	1 (2.7 oz.)	240	2	0	9	21	9.0	60	640	0
smoked, lite	1 (2 oz.)	110	2	0	9	8	3.5	35	530	0
smoked, regular	1 (2 oz.)	190	2	0	7	17	8.0	25	460	0
summer	1 (1 oz.)	88	1	0	4	8	3.5	23	404	0
venison	1 (2 oz.)	177	0	0	7	16	7.0	33	556	0
Vienna	1 (0.6 oz.)	45	0	0	2	4	1.5	8	152	0
Spam®, can										
lite	2 oz.	110	0	0	9	8	3.0	45	560	0
reduced sodium	2 oz.	170	0	0	7	16	6.0	40	560	0
regular	2 oz.	170	0	0	7	16	6.0	40	750	0

MEATS
Specialty & Organ Meats

ITEM	AMOUNT	CALORIES	CARBOHYDRATE (g)	CARBOHYDRATE CHOICES	PROTEIN (g)	FAT (g)	SATURATED FAT (g)	CHOLESTEROL (mg)	SODIUM (mg)	FIBER (g)
Specialty & Organ Meats										
Brains, pan fried	3 oz.	167	0	0	11	13	3.0	1697	134	0
Chitterlings, pork	3 oz.	258	0	0	9	24	8.5	122	33	0
Frog legs	3 oz.	90	0	0	20	0	0.0	62	71	0
Heart	3 oz.	149	0	0	24	5	1.5	164	54	0
Liver, pan fried	3 oz.	185	7	½	23	7	2.5	410	90	0
Oxtail	3 oz.	207	0	0	26	11	5.0	94	162	0
Pigs' feet, pickled	3 oz.	173	0	0	11	14	5.0	78	785	0
Sweetbreads	1 oz.	66	0	0	6	4	2.0	113	15	0
Tongue	3 oz.	241	0	0	19	18	7.5	91	51	0
Tripe	3 oz.	83	0	0	12	3	2.0	81	39	0

MILK & YOGURT
Milk & Milk Beverages

ITEM	AMOUNT	CALORIES	CARBOHYDRATE (g)	CARBOHYDRATE CHOICES	PROTEIN (g)	FAT (g)	SATURATED FAT (g)	CHOLESTEROL (mg)	SODIUM (mg)	FIBER (g)
Acidophilus milk										
1%	1 cup	102	12	1	8	3	1.5	10	123	0
2%	1 cup	130	12	1	8	5	3.0	20	125	0
skim	1 cup	90	13	1	8	0	0.0	5	125	0
Buttermilk										
dried	1 T.	29	4	0	3	0	0.0	5	39	0
lowfat	1 cup	110	12	1	8	3	1.5	15	400	0
skim	1 cup	99	12	1	8	2	1.5	9	257	0
Chocolate milk										
skim	1 cup	144	27	2	9	1	0.5	4	121	1
whole	1 cup	209	26	2	8	9	5.5	31	149	2
Coconut milk, can										
lite	¼ cup	53	1	0	1	5	3.0	0	60	0
regular	¼ cup	90	1	0	1	9	7.0	0	10	0
Condensed milk, sweetened, can										
chocolate	2 T.	120	22	1½	2	3	1.5	10	70	0
fat free	2 T.	110	24	1½	3	0	0.0	0	40	0
whole	2 T.	123	21	1½	3	3	2.0	13	49	0
Eggnog, non-alcoholic										
1 %	1 cup	189	17	1	12	8	4.0	194	155	0
whole	1 cup	343	34	2	10	19	11.0	149	138	0
Evaporated milk, can										
lowfat	½ cup	100	12	1	8	3	2.5	20	139	0
skim	½ cup	99	15	1	10	0	0.0	5	147	0
whole	½ cup	169	13	1	9	10	6.0	37	134	0
Filled milk	1 cup	153	12	1	8	8	7.5	4	138	0
Goat milk	1 cup	168	11	1	9	10	6.5	28	122	0
Human milk	1 fl. oz.	22	2	0	0	1	0.5	4	5	0

MILK & YOGURT
Milk & Milk Beverages

ITEM	AMOUNT	CALORIES	CARBOHYDRATE (g)	CARBOHYDRATE CHOICES	PROTEIN (g)	FAT (g)	SATURATED FAT (g)	CHOLESTEROL (mg)	SODIUM (mg)	FIBER (g)
Instant Breakfast™										
no added sugar, mix, dry	1 pkt.	70	12	1	4	1	0.5	0	95	1
regular, can	1 (10 fl. oz.)	220	37	2½	12	3	1.0	10	70	0
regular, mix, dry	1 pkt.	130	27	2	7	0	0.0	0	134	0
regular, prepared, w/ 1%	1 cup	232	39	2½	15	3	2.0	10	257	0
Kefir										
1%, flavored	1 cup	160	28	2	8	2	1.5	15	120	0
1%, plain	1 cup	110	13	1	8	2	1.5	15	125	0
2%, plain	1 cup	122	9	½	9	5	3.0	10	50	0
Lactaid® milk										
lowfat	1 cup	130	12	1	8	5	3.0	20	125	0
skim	1 cup	80	13	1	8	0	0.0	0	125	0
Lowfat milk										
1 %	1 cup	102	12	1	8	3	1.5	10	123	0
1%, protein fortified	1 cup	119	14	1	10	3	2.0	10	143	0
2 %	1 cup	121	12	1	8	5	3.0	18	122	0
Malted milk drink	1 cup	228	30	2	9	9	6.0	34	172	1
Milk shake, w/ whole	1 cup	288	46	3	8	8	5.0	29	220	0
Ovaltine®, w/ skim	1 cup	170	30	2	10	0	0.0	5	185	0
Powdered milk, dry										
nonfat	¼ cup	61	9	½	6	0	0.0	3	93	0
whole	¼ cup	159	12	1	8	9	5.0	31	119	0
Rice Dream® beverage										
1%, plain	1 cup	120	25	1½	1	2	0.0	0	90	0
1%, vanilla flavored	1 cup	130	28	2	1	2	0.0	0	90	0
Sheep milk	1 cup	265	13	1	15	17	11.5	66	108	0
Skim milk	1 cup	86	12	1	8	0	0.0	4	126	0
Soy beverage										
1%, plain	1 cup	100	15	1	3	2	0.5	0	120	0
1%, vanilla	1 cup	120	21	1½	3	3	0.5	0	120	0
regular, plain	1 cup	160	14	1	9	7	1.0	0	180	0
Sport Shake®, can	1 (11 fl. oz.)	430	63	4	13	13	8.0	55	310	0
Strawberry Milk, Quik®	1 cup	230	33	2	7	8	5.0	30	100	0
Veggie Milk®	1 cup	110	13	1	9	3	0.0	0	90	2
Whole milk	1 cup	150	11	1	8	8	5.0	33	120	0
Yogurt										
Flavored										
fat free, w/ aspartame	1 cup	100	18	1	8	0	0.0	5	115	0
lowfat, fruited	1 cup	232	43	3	10	2	1.5	10	133	0
lowfat, w/ topping	6 oz.	180	35	2	7	1	0.5	5	115	0
Plain										
fat free	1 cup	100	19	1	10	0	0.0	5	135	0

MILK & YOGURT
Yogurt

ITEM	AMOUNT	CALORIES	CARBOHYDRATE (g)	CARBOHYDRATE CHOICES	PROTEIN (g)	FAT (g)	SATURATED FAT (g)	CHOLESTEROL (mg)	SODIUM (mg)	FIBER (g)
Plain *(con't.)*										
lowfat	1 cup	110	13	1	9	2	1.5	10	135	0
whole milk	1 cup	180	12	1	9	10	6.0	40	125	0
Soy										
lowfat, plain	1 cup	140	21	1½	8	3	0.0	0	10	0
whole milk, flavored	1 cup	247	33	2	12	8	5.0	24	158	0
whole milk, plain	1 cup	150	11	1	9	8	5.0	31	114	0
Yo-J™	1 cup	150	35	2	3	0	0.0	0	55	0

NUTS, SEEDS & PEANUT BUTTER

ITEM	AMOUNT	CALORIES	CARBOHYDRATE (g)	CARBOHYDRATE CHOICES	PROTEIN (g)	FAT (g)	SATURATED FAT (g)	CHOLESTEROL (mg)	SODIUM (mg)	FIBER (g)
Almond butter	1 T.	99	3	0	2	9	1.0	0	70	1
Almond paste	1 T.	65	7	½	1	4	0.0	0	1	1
Almonds	24	166	7	½	5	15	1.0	0	3	3
Beechnuts	10	184	4	0	7	17	0.0	0	0	1
Brazilnuts	8	186	4	0	4	19	5.0	0	1	2
Cashew butter	1 T.	94	4	0	3	8	1.5	0	98	0
Cashews, salted	18	163	9	½	4	13	3.0	0	120	1
Chestnuts	3	69	15	1	1	1	0.0	0	1	2
Filberts/hazelnuts	30	179	4	0	4	18	1.0	0	1	2
Flax seeds	2 T.	95	7	0	4	7	0.5	0	7	5
Hickory nuts	10	197	5	0	4	19	2.0	0	0	2
Macadamias	12	199	4	0	2	21	3.0	0	1	2
Mixed nuts										
w/ peanuts, salted	28	168	7	½	5	15	2.0	0	110	3
w/o peanuts, salted	20	174	6	½	4	16	3.0	0	110	2
Peanut butter										
chunky/creamy	1 T.	94	3	0	4	8	2.0	0	78	1
natural	1 T.	93	3	0	4	8	1.0	0	40	1
reduced fat	1 T.	95	8	½	4	6	1.0	0	95	1
Peanuts										
Beer nuts®	39	170	7	½	7	14	3.0	0	80	2
dry roasted, salted	39	160	6	½	7	13	2.0	0	190	2
honey roasted	39	160	8	½	6	13	1.5	0	95	2
Sweet N' Crunchy®	18	140	16	1	4	7	1.0	0	20	2
w/ oil, salted	39	170	5	0	7	15	2.5	0	130	2
Pecans	31	189	5	0	2	19	2.0	0	0	1
Pine nuts	¼ cup	180	9	½	4	14	3.0	0	0	3
Pistachio nuts	47	164	7	½	6	14	2.0	0	2	3
Poppy seeds	1 T.	47	2	0	2	4	0.5	0	2	1
Pumpkin/squash seeds	2 T.	93	4	0	3	8	1.0	0	0	1
Sesame butter/tahini	1 T.	91	3	0	3	8	1.0	0	0	1
Sesame seeds	2 T.	103	4	0	3	9	1.0	0	2	2

NUTS, SEEDS & PEANUT BUTTER

ITEM	AMOUNT	CALORIES	CARBOHYDRATE (g)	CARBOHYDRATE CHOICES	PROTEIN (g)	FAT (g)	SATURATED FAT (g)	CHOLESTEROL (mg)	SODIUM (mg)	FIBER (g)
Soynut butter	1 T.	85	5	0	4	6	1.0	0	58	1
Soynuts, salted	¼ cup	127	9	0	10	7	1.0	0	164	8
Sunflower seeds, salted	2 T.	104	2	0	4	10	1.0	0	102	1
Trail mix										
w/ chocolate chips	¼ cup	137	13	1	4	9	2.0	1	34	2
w/ fruit, tropical	¼ cup	115	19	1	2	5	2.0	0	3	2
w/ seeds	¼ cup	131	13	1	4	8	1.5	0	65	2
Walnuts, chopped	2 T.	95	2	0	4	9	0.5	0	0	1

PASTA, RICE & OTHER GRAINS
Cooked unless indicated
Pasta

ITEM	AMOUNT	CALORIES	CARBOHYDRATE (g)	CARBOHYDRATE CHOICES	PROTEIN (g)	FAT (g)	SATURATED FAT (g)	CHOLESTEROL (mg)	SODIUM (mg)	FIBER (g)
Cellophane noodles	1 cup	210	51	3½	0	0	0.0	0	14	0
Chinese noodles	1 cup	300	68	4½	10	2	0.0	0	0	2
Chow mein noodles, can	1 cup	280	36	2½	6	14	3.0	0	420	0
Egg noodles	1 cup	213	40	2½	8	2	0.5	53	11	2
Gnocchi	1 cup	272	33	2	5	14	8.5	37	142	2
Macaroni	1 cup	197	40	2½	7	1	0.0	0	1	2
Macaroni, whole wheat	1 cup	174	37	2½	7	0	0.0	0	4	4
Pasta & sauce, mix										
cheddar broccoli	1 cup	260	46	3	9	4	1.5	10	870	1
garlic & butter	1 cup	210	40	2½	7	3	1.0	5	780	2
three cheese	1 cup	240	41	3	9	5	3.0	10	870	1
Pasta Roni®, box										
fettucini Alfredo	1 cup	460	49	3	12	25	6.0	10	1150	2
herb & butter	1 cup	380	42	3	10	19	4.5	5	960	2
shells & cheddar	1 cup	310	40	2½	9	13	3.5	5	730	2
Ramen noodles, w/ seasoning	1 cup	190	26	2	4	8	4.0	0	900	1
Ravioli, cheese	1 cup	290	38	2½	14	9	5.0	70	340	3
Rice noodles	1 cup	160	39	2½	0	0	0.0	0	9	0
Soba noodles	1 cup	113	24	1½	6	0	0.0	0	68	1
Spaghetti	1 cup	197	40	2½	7	1	0.0	0	1	2
Tortellini										
w/ cheese	1 cup	347	49	3	16	8	4.5	40	307	1
w/ meat	1 cup	372	33	2	24	15	5.5	238	797	1

Rice

ITEM	AMOUNT	CALORIES	CARBOHYDRATE (g)	CARBOHYDRATE CHOICES	PROTEIN (g)	FAT (g)	SATURATED FAT (g)	CHOLESTEROL (mg)	SODIUM (mg)	FIBER (g)
Basmati	½ cup	80	18	1	2	0	0.0	0	5	0
Brown	½ cup	108	22	1½	3	1	0.0	0	5	2
Fried	½ cup	132	17	1	3	6	1.0	21	143	1
Pilaf	½ cup	85	18	1	3	0	0.0	0	0	1
Rice A Roni®, chicken										
reduced sodium	½ cup	140	27	2	4	3	0.5	0	340	1

PASTA, RICE & OTHER GRAINS

Rice

ITEM	AMOUNT	CALORIES	CARBOHYDRATE (g)	CARBOHYDRATE CHOICES	PROTEIN (g)	FAT (g)	SATURATED FAT (g)	CHOLESTEROL (mg)	SODIUM (mg)	FIBER (g)
Rice A Roni®, chicken *(con't.)*										
regular	½ cup	155	26	2	4	5	1.0	0	545	1
Risotto	½ cup	281	29	2	7	15	9.0	36	851	1
Spanish	½ cup	108	21	1½	2	2	0.5	0	162	2
White										
instant	½ cup	81	18	1	2	0	0.0	0	2	0
regular	½ cup	133	29	2	3	0	0.0	0	1	1
Wild	½ cup	83	17	1	3	0	0.0	0	2	1
Other Grains										
Barley										
pearled	½ cup	97	22	1½	2	0	0.0	0	2	3
whole	½ cup	135	30	1½	4	1	0.0	0	1	7
Buckwheat/kasha	½ cup	77	17	1	3	1	0.0	0	3	2
Bulgur	½ cup	76	17	1	3	0	0.0	0	5	4
Couscous	1 cup	200	42	3	6	0	0.0	0	8	2
Millet	½ cup	143	28	2	4	1	0.0	0	2	2
Polenta										
fried, slice	1 (4 oz.)	168	30	2	4	4	0.0	0	530	2
w/ milk	½ cup	163	21	1½	4	8	3.0	12	571	2
Quinoa	½ cup	150	28	2	5	2	0.0	0	0	4

POULTRY

Cooked w/o fat unless indicated

Chicken

ITEM	AMOUNT	CALORIES	CARBOHYDRATE (g)	CARBOHYDRATE CHOICES	PROTEIN (g)	FAT (g)	SATURATED FAT (g)	CHOLESTEROL (mg)	SODIUM (mg)	FIBER (g)
Breasts										
BBQ, w/ skin	3 oz.	163	2	0	20	8	2.0	62	177	0
breaded & fried, w/ skin	3 oz.	221	8	½	21	11	3.0	72	234	0
deli	1 oz.	45	1	0	6	2	0.5	14	166	0
fried, w/ skin	3 oz.	189	1	0	27	8	2.0	76	65	0
fried, w/o skin	3 oz.	159	0	0	28	4	1.0	77	67	0
roasted, w/ skin	3 oz.	168	0	0	25	7	2.0	71	60	0
roasted, w/o skin	3 oz.	140	0	0	26	3	1.0	72	63	0
Capon, roasted, w/ skin	3 oz.	195	0	0	25	10	3.0	73	42	0
Cornish hens										
roasted, w/ skin	3 oz.	202	0	0	23	12	3.0	74	266	0
roasted, w/o skin	3 oz.	161	0	0	24	6	1.5	75	269	0
Fingers, fried	6	290	15	1	18	17	3.5	60	510	0
Giblets, fried	3 oz.	236	4	0	28	11	3.0	379	96	0
Gizzards, simmered	3 oz.	130	1	0	23	3	1.0	165	57	0
Hearts, simmered	3 oz.	157	0	0	22	7	2.0	206	41	0
Hot dogs	1 (1.6 oz.)	116	3	0	6	9	2.5	45	617	0

POULTRY
Chicken

ITEM	AMOUNT	CALORIES	CARBOHYDRATE (g)	CARBOHYDRATE CHOICES	PROTEIN (g)	FAT (g)	SATURATED FAT (g)	CHOLESTEROL (mg)	SODIUM (mg)	FIBER (g)
Legs										
breaded & fried, w/ skin	3 oz.	232	7	½	19	14	3.5	77	237	0
fried, w/ skin	3 oz.	216	2	0	23	12	3.5	80	75	0
fried, w/o skin	3 oz.	177	1	0	24	8	2.0	84	82	0
roasted, w/ skin	3 oz.	197	0	0	22	11	3.0	78	74	0
roasted, w/o skin	3 oz.	146	0	0	24	5	1.5	79	81	0
Livers	3 oz.	134	1	0	21	5	1.5	537	43	0
Pâté, chicken liver, can	1 oz.	57	2	0	4	4	1.0	111	109	0
Patties, breaded & fried	1 (3 oz.)	242	13	1	14	15	5.0	51	452	0
Thighs										
breaded & fried, w/ skin	3 oz.	248	9	½	17	15	4.0	95	434	0
fried, w/ skin	3 oz.	223	3	0	23	13	3.5	83	75	0
fried, w/o skin	3 oz.	185	1	0	24	9	2.0	87	81	0
roasted, w/ skin	3 oz.	210	0	0	21	13	3.5	79	71	0
roasted, w/o skin	3 oz.	166	0	0	21	8	2.5	77	64	0
Wings										
fried, w/ skin	1	103	1	0	8	7	2.0	26	25	0
roasted, w/ skin	1	99	0	0	9	7	2.0	29	28	0
Game										
Duck										
roasted, w/ skin	3 oz.	287	0	0	16	24	8.0	71	50	0
roasted, w/o skin	3 oz.	171	0	0	20	10	3.5	76	55	0
Goose										
roasted, w/ skin	3 oz.	259	0	0	21	19	6.0	77	60	0
roasted, w/o skin	3 oz.	202	0	0	25	11	4.0	82	65	0
Ostrich										
ground	3 oz.	121	0	0	23	3	1.0	71	64	0
tenderloin	3 oz.	113	0	0	20	3	1.0	81	61	0
Pheasant										
roasted, w/ skin	3 oz.	207	0	0	26	11	3.0	81	46	0
roasted, w/o skin	3 oz.	151	0	0	27	4	1.5	75	42	0
Quail										
roasted, w/ skin	3 oz.	218	0	0	22	14	4.0	86	60	0
roasted, w/o skin	3 oz.	152	0	0	25	5	1.5	79	58	0
Turkey										
Bacon	2 slices	68	1	0	4	5	1.5	24	368	0
Bologna	1 oz.	56	0	0	4	4	1.5	28	249	0
Breast, deli	1 oz.	31	0	0	6	0	0.0	12	406	0
Dark meat										
roasted, w/ skin	3 oz.	184	0	0	23	9	3.0	77	68	0
roasted, w/o skin	3 oz.	157	0	0	24	6	2.0	75	70	0

POULTRY
Turkey

ITEM	AMOUNT	CALORIES	CARBOHYDRATE (g)	CARBOHYDRATE CHOICES	PROTEIN (g)	FAT (g)	SATURATED FAT (g)	CHOLESTEROL (mg)	SODIUM (mg)	FIBER (g)
Ground										
extra lean	3 oz.	120	0	0	27	2	0.5	55	75	0
lean	3 oz.	169	0	0	20	9	2.5	90	107	0
Ham, deli	1 oz.	37	0	0	5	2	0.5	19	275	0
Hot dogs	1 (1.6 oz.)	102	1	0	6	8	2.5	48	642	0
Light meat										
roasted, w/ skin	3 oz.	139	0	0	24	4	1.0	81	48	0
roasted, w/o skin	3 oz.	119	0	0	26	1	0.0	73	48	0
Pastrami, deli	1 oz.	40	0	0	5	2	0.5	15	296	0
Patties, breaded & fried	1 (3 oz.)	241	13	1	12	15	4.0	53	680	0
Sausages	1 (2 oz.)	93	0	0	11	6	1.5	43	470	0

RESTAURANT FAVORITES
Appetizers

ITEM	AMOUNT	CALORIES	CARBOHYDRATE (g)	CARBOHYDRATE CHOICES	PROTEIN (g)	FAT (g)	SATURATED FAT (g)	CHOLESTEROL (mg)	SODIUM (mg)	FIBER (g)
Breadsticks	1 medium	140	26	2	5	2	0.0	0	270	1
Bruschetta	1 (4 in.)	62	6	½	2	4	1.0	2	125	0
Buffalo wings	4	210	4	0	22	12	3.0	130	900	0
Clams casino	6	377	19	1	35	17	10.0	115	802	1
Crab cakes, fried	1 (4 oz.)	290	20	1	9	19	4.0	149	893	0
Cream cheese puffs	3	331	14	1	3	29	6.5	18	180	0
Focaccia bread	1 (6 in.)	271	47	3	7	6	1.0	0	446	3
Garlic bread	1 (4 in.)	322	38	2½	12	14	4.0	20	522	4
Jalapeño poppers	6	360	32	2	7	22	10.0	45	810	3
Mozzarella sticks, w/ sauce	4	378	28	2	19	22	12.0	24	2712	3
Mushrooms, fried	8	237	13	1	4	19	3.0	22	193	1
Nachos, deluxe	1 order	1048	91	5	46	57	23.0	109	2252	17
Oysters Rockefeller	6	170	10	½	8	10	2.0	46	392	0
Pork dumplings, fried	1 (3.5 oz.)	340	24	1½	13	21	6.0	29	346	1
Potato skins	6	500	30	1½	20	34	14.0	80	1020	8
Shrimp cocktail, w/ sauce	5	42	3	0	6	0	0.0	54	262	0
Spring rolls, w/ meat	1 (2.5 oz.)	127	10	½	6	7	2.0	41	336	1
Stuffed mushrooms	3	134	10	½	4	9	5.0	23	183	1
Wontons, w/ meat	1 (0.7 oz.)	61	4	0	3	4	0.5	13	83	0
Beverages										
Bahama Mama	6 fl. oz.	288	21	1½	1	1	1.0	0	31	0
Café latte										
w/ skim milk	12 fl. oz.	120	20	1	13	1	0.0	5	170	0
w/ whole milk	12 fl. oz.	210	19	1	12	11	7.0	45	170	0
w/ whole milk, flavored	12 fl. oz.	258	29	2	11	11	7.0	45	160	0
Café mocha										
w/ skim milk, w/ whipped cream	12 fl. oz.	260	36	2½	14	12	6.5	43	160	0

RESTAURANT FAVORITES
Beverages

ITEM	AMOUNT	CALORIES	CARBOHYDRATE (g)	CARBOHYDRATE CHOICES	PROTEIN (g)	FAT (g)	SATURATED FAT (g)	CHOLESTEROL (mg)	SODIUM (mg)	FIBER (g)
Café mocha *(con't.)*										
w/ skim milk,										
w/o whipped cream	12 fl. oz.	180	35	2	14	3	1.5	8	150	0
w/ whole milk,										
w/ whipped cream	12 fl. oz.	340	34	2	13	21	13.0	70	160	0
Cappuccino										
w/ skim milk	12 fl. oz.	80	11	1	7	0	0.0	5	110	0
w/ whole milk	12 fl. oz.	140	11	1	7	7	4.5	30	105	0
Colorado Bulldog	4 fl. oz.	248	13	1	1	11	7.0	41	18	0
Espresso	3 fl. oz.	8	1	0	0	0	0.0	0	12	0
Sangria	8 fl. oz.	194	27	2	0	0	0.0	0	17	0
Smoothie	16 fl. oz.	320	70	4½	7	1	0.5	5	160	4
Desserts										
Apple pie à la mode	1 (6 oz.)	433	58	4	5	21	8.0	29	292	2
Caramel apple bars	1 (5 oz.)	370	54	3½	4	18	3.0	25	200	1
Carrot cake, w/ icing	1 (4 oz.)	494	53	3½	5	30	6.0	61	279	1
Cheesecake	1 (3 oz.)	295	23	1½	5	21	11.0	51	190	0
Chocolate chip cookies	1 (2 oz.)	280	40	2½	3	13	8.0	40	85	2
Chocolate mousse cake	1 (3 oz.)	291	41	3	2	12	4.0	29	140	2
Chocolate peanut butter pie	1 (6 oz.)	653	64	4	12	39	19.0	27	319	3
Crème Brûlée	¾ cup	347	35	2	7	20	11.0	311	125	0
Fortune cookies	1	30	7	½	0	0	0.0	0	22	0
Fudge brownie sundae	1 (8 oz.)	687	83	5½	9	38	11.0	62	486	3
Key lime pie	1 (4.5 oz.)	380	58	4	5	14	5.0	15	240	0
Tiramisu	1 (5 oz.)	368	33	2	9	22	13.0	187	291	0
Entrées:										
American										
BBQ beef sandwich	1 (6.5 oz.)	392	39	2½	20	17	6.0	54	1056	3
BBQ pork sandwich	1 (6.5 oz.)	347	39	2½	23	10	3.0	52	889	3
BBQ ribs	8 oz.	700	36	2½	44	42	18.0	130	1240	0
Chicken fried steak	8 oz.	530	28	2	30	34	16.0	54	1336	2
Filet mignon	8 oz.	479	0	0	64	23	8.5	191	143	0
Fried shrimp	12 large	218	10	½	19	11	2.0	159	310	0
Grilled salmon	8 oz.	423	0	0	59	19	3.0	135	265	0
King crab legs	9 oz.	248	0	0	50	4	0.0	135	2735	0
Potato, w/ broccoli & cheese	1 (10 oz.)	1168	114	6½	28	71	18.0	52	1684	16
Prime rib	12 oz.	1334	0	0	74	113	47.0	289	211	0
Shrimp Creole, w/ rice	2 cups	611	51	3½	55	19	4.0	371	1310	3
Shrimp jambalaya	2 cups	611	51	3½	55	19	4.0	371	1310	3
Southwestern tuna wrap	1 (14 oz.)	950	53	3½	41	64	17.0	110	1230	4
Stuffed shrimp	2 cups	552	17	1	56	27	6.0	443	1388	1
T-bone steak	10 oz.	530	0	0	42	40	18.0	121	534	0

RESTAURANT FAVORITES
Entrées: American

ITEM	AMOUNT	CALORIES	CARBOHYDRATE (g)	CARBOHYDRATE CHOICES	PROTEIN (g)	FAT (g)	SATURATED FAT (g)	CHOLESTEROL (mg)	SODIUM (mg)	FIBER (g)
Turkey & cheese bagel	1 (11 oz.)	506	66	4½	34	11	5.5	56	1393	4
Asian/Chinese										
Beef & broccoli	2 cups	512	14	½	76	39	10.0	202	1473	5
Cashew chicken	2 cups	817	23	1½	54	57	9.5	121	1975	4
Chicken curry	2 cups	586	20	1	54	32	7.0	168	2376	4
Egg rolls, meatless	1 (2.5 oz.)	113	11	1	3	6	1.5	33	339	1
Kung Pao chicken	2 cups	818	22	1½	54	58	10.0	120	1976	4
Pork chow mein, w/ noodles	2 cups	869	62	3½	44	51	10.5	96	1631	7
Shrimp & snow peas	2 cups	439	19	1	38	23	3.0	295	2134	3
Stir-fry chicken & fried rice	2 cups	432	45	3	19	19	3.5	85	853	3
Sushi, w/ fish & vegetables	1 cup	238	48	3	9	1	0.0	11	344	1
Sweet & sour pork, w/ rice	2 cups	537	79	5	26	13	3.5	57	1813	3
Tofu & vegetable stir-fry	2 cups	293	34	1½	15	14	2.0	0	445	10
Italian/Mediterranean										
Calzones, w/ pepperoni	1 (6 oz.)	450	49	3	21	19	9.0	10	930	6
Chicken cacciatore	2 cups	916	26	2	84	51	13.0	320	1183	4
Chicken cordon bleu	8 oz.	483	9	½	46	28	15.0	191	489	1
Chicken Marsala	8 oz.	593	12	1	55	31	11.0	177	540	1
Chicken/veal parmigiana	8 oz.	466	29	2	36	23	8.0	115	929	1
Eggs Benedict	19 oz.	860	55	3½	35	56	23.0	525	1943	3
Fettuccini Alfredo	2 cups	1430	68	4½	31	119	71.0	340	1470	3
Gyros	½ pita	296	23	1½	15	15	7.5	55	604	1
Linguini, w/ pesto sauce	2 cups	706	83	5	23	31	7.0	18	425	6
Lobster Newburg	2 cups	1225	23	1½	60	100	59.0	738	1294	0
Moussaka	2 cups	474	26	1	33	26	9.0	193	863	7
Pasta, w/ carbonara sauce	2 cups	651	83	5	25	24	10.5	93	496	5
Pasta, w/ marinara sauce	2 cups	530	94	5½	17	9	1.0	0	1100	10
Seafood Alfredo	2 cups	1014	62	4	38	69	41.0	337	672	5
Shrimp scampi	2 cups	438	2	0	58	20	10.0	480	584	0
Spanakopita	8 oz.	387	37	2½	16	20	10.0	227	769	4
Stuffed grape leaves	4	212	7	½	7	17	4.0	52	65	1
Veal scallopini	8 oz.	608	2	0	42	46	13.0	146	900	0
Vegetarian lasagna	2 cups	720	70	4½	40	34	24.0	130	1740	4
Mexican										
Chimichangas, beef & cheese	1 (6.5 oz.)	443	39	2½	20	23	11.0	51	957	0
Enchiladas										
cheese	2 (6 in.)	639	57	4	19	38	21.0	88	1568	1
seafood	2 (6 in.)	529	43	3	25	29	17.0	83	1372	1
Fajitas										
chicken	1 (9 oz.)	520	53	3½	18	26	8.0	70	1300	4
steak	1 (9 oz.)	510	52	3½	21	25	8.0	50	1200	3
Huevos rancheros	1 (2 egg)	410	24	1½	23	26	9.5	450	530	4

RESTAURANT FAVORITES
Entrées: Mexican

ITEM	AMOUNT	CALORIES	CARBOHYDRATE (g)	CARBOHYDRATE CHOICES	PROTEIN (g)	FAT (g)	SATURATED FAT (g)	CHOLESTEROL (mg)	SODIUM (mg)	FIBER (g)
Quesadillas	1 (2 oz.)	199	21	1½	6	10	3.5	14	255	1
Rice & beans	2 cups	520	84	5	20	12	4.0	20	1440	12
Salads, w/ dressing										
Caesar	4 cups	338	20	1	8	25	5.0	7	725	3
Chicken Caesar	4 cups	655	23	1½	37	47	9.0	86	1728	4
Greek	1 (14 oz.)	441	18	1	13	37	14.0	67	1301	4
Niçoise	1 (12 oz.)	423	26	1½	19	28	4.0	36	1026	5
Oriental chicken	1 (9 oz.)	270	17	1	40	4	0.5	70	700	5
Tossed, w/ Gorgonzola	4 cups	400	9	½	20	34	13.0	50	800	3
Side Dishes										
Garlic mashed potatoes	1 cup	209	18	1	3	14	8.0	33	132	3
Grilled vegetables	1½ cups	120	15	1	6	4	0.0	0	310	3
Oven roasted potatoes	1½ cups	260	50	3	6	6	1.0	0	300	4
Polenta	½ cup	163	21	1½	4	8	3.0	12	571	2
Ratatouille	1 cup	133	12	1	2	10	1.5	0	106	4
Risotto	½ cup	281	29	2	7	15	9.0	36	851	1
Soft pretzels	1 large	340	72	5	10	1	0.0	0	900	3
Soups										
Borscht	1 cup	73	7	½	3	4	2.5	8	498	2
Cheese	1 cup	626	28	2	36	42	26.0	132	1464	2
Chicken chili	1 cup	233	21	1½	14	12	7.0	43	1353	4
Chilled fruit	1 cup	99	25	1½	1	0	0.0	0	12	1
Clam chowder	1 cup	270	16	1	11	20	9.0	63	730	1
Egg drop	1 cup	73	1	0	8	4	1.0	103	729	0
French onion, w/ croutons	1 cup	260	27	2	12	12	6.0	18	1020	2
Gazpacho	1 cup	68	10	½	2	3	0.0	0	286	2
Hot & sour	1 cup	133	5	0	12	6	2.0	23	1563	0
Minestrone	1 cup	154	23	1½	6	5	0.5	0	790	4
Seafood stew	1 cup	173	9	½	23	5	1.0	95	359	2
Shrimp gumbo	1 cup	151	18	1	10	5	1.0	50	590	4
Tomato Florentine	1 cup	61	14	1	4	1	0.5	3	1035	3
Vichyssoise	1 cup	223	18	1	5	15	8.0	44	336	2
Wonton	1 cup	45	5	0	4	1	0.0	15	940	1

SALAD DRESSINGS

ITEM	AMOUNT	CALORIES	CARBOHYDRATE (g)	CARBOHYDRATE CHOICES	PROTEIN (g)	FAT (g)	SATURATED FAT (g)	CHOLESTEROL (mg)	SODIUM (mg)	FIBER (g)
Bacon & tomato										
light	1 T.	32	0	0	0	3	0.5	1	176	0
regular	1 T.	65	4	0	0	6	0.5	0	205	0
Blue cheese										
fat free	1 T.	25	6	½	0	0	0.0	0	170	1
light	1 T.	40	1	0	1	4	1.0	0	190	0
regular	1 T.	77	1	0	1	8	1.5	3	168	0

SALAD DRESSINGS

ITEM	AMOUNT	CALORIES	CARBOHYDRATE (g)	CARBOHYDRATE CHOICES	PROTEIN (g)	FAT (g)	SATURATED FAT (g)	CHOLESTEROL (mg)	SODIUM (mg)	FIBER (g)
Buttermilk	1 T.	75	1	0	0	8	1.5	1	115	0
Caesar										
fat free	1 T.	5	1	0	0	0	0.0	0	195	0
light	1 T.	17	3	0	0	1	0.0	0	162	0
regular	1 T.	65	1	0	1	7	1.5	1	185	0
Catalina®										
fat free	1 T.	18	4	0	0	0	0.0	0	160	0
regular	1 T.	70	4	0	0	6	1.0	0	195	0
Creamy cucumber										
light	1 T.	24	1	0	0	2	0.0	0	153	0
regular	1 T.	60	2	0	0	6	0.5	3	130	0
Creamy garlic	1 T.	80	1	0	0	9	0.5	3	115	0
Creamy Parmesan	1 T.	85	1	0	0	9	1.0	5	130	0
French										
fat free	1 T.	20	6	½	0	0	0.0	0	150	0
light	1 T.	22	4	0	0	1	0.0	0	128	0
regular	1 T.	67	3	0	0	6	1.5	0	214	0
Garlic & herb										
creamy	1 T.	55	1	0	0	6	1.0	0	175	0
regular, mix, prepared	1 T.	70	1	0	0	8	1.0	0	170	0
Green Goddess®	1 T.	60	1	0	0	7	1.0	0	130	0
Honey mustard	1 T.	75	2	0	0	8	1.0	0	120	0
Italian										
creamy	1 T.	55	2	0	0	6	2.0	1	115	0
fat free	1 T.	5	1	0	0	0	0.0	0	145	0
light	1 T.	16	1	0	0	1	0.0	1	118	0
pesto	1 T.	35	3	0	0	5	0.5	0	130	0
regular	1 T.	69	2	0	0	7	1.0	0	116	0
regular, mix, prepared	1 T.	70	1	0	0	8	1.0	0	160	0
Oil & vinegar	1 T.	72	0	0	0	8	1.0	0	0	0
Ranch										
fat free	1 T.	25	6	½	0	0	0.0	0	155	0
light	1 T.	50	4	0	1	4	1.0	3	120	0
regular	1 T.	85	1	0	0	9	1.5	3	135	0
Russian										
light	1 T.	23	5	0	0	1	0.0	1	141	0
regular	1 T.	76	2	0	0	8	1.0	3	133	0
Sesame seed	1 T.	68	1	0	0	7	1.0	0	153	0
Thousand island										
fat free	1 T.	23	6	½	0	0	0.0	0	150	1
light	1 T.	40	4	0	0	3	0.5	5	125	0
regular	1 T.	55	3	0	0	5	1.0	5	155	0

SALAD DRESSINGS

ITEM	AMOUNT	CALORIES	CARBOHYDRATE (g)	CARBOHYDRATE CHOICES	PROTEIN (g)	FAT (g)	SATURATED FAT (g)	CHOLESTEROL (mg)	SODIUM (mg)	FIBER (g)
Vinaigrette, red wine										
fat free	1 T.	8	2	0	0	0	0.0	0	200	0
light	1 T.	23	2	0	0	4	0.0	0	160	0
regular	1 T.	69	2	0	0	8	1.0	0	116	0
Western®										
light	1 T.	35	6	½	0	2	0.0	0	135	0
regular	1 T.	75	6	½	0	6	1.0	0	120	0

For mayonnaise/Miracle Whip®
see Fats, Oils, Cream & Gravy

SALADS

ITEM	AMOUNT	CALORIES	CARBOHYDRATE (g)	CARBOHYDRATE CHOICES	PROTEIN (g)	FAT (g)	SATURATED FAT (g)	CHOLESTEROL (mg)	SODIUM (mg)	FIBER (g)
Caesar, w/ dressing	1 cup	200	7	½	7	17	4.5	15	450	1
Carrot-raisin	½ cup	202	21	1½	1	14	2.0	10	117	2
Chef										
w/ dressing	1 cup	312	9	½	17	23	7.5	111	924	2
w/o dressing	1 cup	178	3	0	17	11	5.5	93	496	2
Chicken, w/ mayo.	½ cup	268	1	0	11	25	3.0	48	201	0
Coleslaw										
w/ mayo.	½ cup	98	9	½	1	7	1.0	3	178	1
w/ vinaigrette	½ cup	41	7	½	1	2	0.0	5	14	1
Cucumber										
creamy, w/ mayo.	½ cup	59	5	0	1	4	3.0	9	13	1
w/ vinegar	½ cup	24	6	½	0	0	0.0	0	175	1
Egg, w/ mayo.	½ cup	293	1	0	8	28	5.0	287	333	0
Fruit, fresh	½ cup	51	13	1	1	0	0.0	0	0	1
Gelatin, w/ fruit	½ cup	73	18	1	1	0	0.0	0	30	1
Ham, w/ mayo.	½ cup	259	13	1	10	19	6.0	44	1094	0
Lobster, w/ mayo.	½ cup	69	5	0	5	3	0.5	50	263	1
Macaroni, w/ mayo.	½ cup	230	14	1	2	19	2.0	14	176	1
Pasta primavera	½ cup	189	19	1	4	11	2.0	0	386	2
Potato										
German style	½ cup	106	18	1	2	3	3.0	4	318	2
w/ eggs & mayo.	½ cup	179	14	1	3	10	2.0	85	661	2
w/ mayo.	½ cup	133	16	1	2	7	1.0	5	344	2
Seafood										
w/ mayo.	½ cup	166	2	0	12	12	1.5	64	274	0
w/ pasta, vinaigrette	½ cup	126	11	1	5	7	1.0	17	524	1
Shrimp, w/ mayo.	½ cup	141	3	0	13	8	1.5	103	195	0
Spinach, w/o dressing	1 cup	89	10	½	4	4	1.0	61	157	2
Suddenly Salad®, box										
Caesar	¾ cup	220	3	0	5	1	0.0	0	580	1
classic	¾ cup	250	38	2½	7	2	0.0	0	910	2

SALADS

ITEM	AMOUNT	CALORIES	CARBOHYDRATE (g)	CARBOHYDRATE CHOICES	PROTEIN (g)	FAT (g)	SATURATED FAT (g)	CHOLESTEROL (mg)	SODIUM (mg)	FIBER (g)
Suddenly Salad®, box *(con't.)*										
garden Italian	¾ cup	140	28	2	5	1	0.0	0	520	2
Tabbouleh	½ cup	120	12	1	4	4	0.0	0	252	3
Taco										
w/ salsa	1 (17 oz.)	420	32	1	24	22	11.0	60	1520	15
w/ salsa & shell	1 (19 oz.)	850	65	3	30	52	15.0	60	1780	16
Three bean, w/ oil	½ cup	82	17	1	4	4	0.5	0	202	5
Tortellini, cheese	½ cup	164	18	1	4	8	2.0	7	564	2
Tossed, w/o dressing	1 cup	25	5	0	1	0	0.0	0	15	2
Tuna, w/ mayo.	½ cup	192	10	½	16	10	1.5	13	412	0
Waldorf, w/ mayo.	½ cup	204	6	½	2	20	2.0	10	118	1

SOUPS

Canned, prepared

ITEM	AMOUNT	CALORIES	CARBOHYDRATE (g)	CARBOHYDRATE CHOICES	PROTEIN (g)	FAT (g)	SATURATED FAT (g)	CHOLESTEROL (mg)	SODIUM (mg)	FIBER (g)
Bean										
w/ bacon	1 cup	180	25	1	8	5	2.0	0	890	7
w/ franks	1 cup	188	22	1	10	7	2.0	130	1093	6
Beef barley, w/ veg.	1 cup	130	13	1	10	4	1.5	25	780	3
Beef broth										
reduced sodium	1 cup	38	1	0	5	1	0.0	0	72	0
regular	1 cup	20	2	0	2	1	0.0	0	1010	0
Beef consommé	1 cup	25	2	0	4	0	0.0	0	820	0
Beef noodle	1 cup	89	9	½	5	3	1.0	5	952	1
Black bean	1 cup	170	30	1	8	1.5	0.0	3	730	10
Cheddar cheese*	1 cup	181	17	1	8	9	4.5	25	1142	1
Chicken alphabet	1 cup	80	11	1	4	2	1.0	10	880	1
Chicken & dumplings	1 cup	96	6	½	6	6	1.0	34	860	1
Chicken & rice	1 cup	110	12	1	7	3	1.0	15	750	1
Chicken broth										
reduced sodium	1 cup	15	1	0	3	0	0.0	0	620	0
regular	1 cup	30	1	0	2	2	0.0	0	1000	0
Chicken gumbo	1 cup	56	8	½	3	1	0.0	5	954	2
Chicken noodle	1 cup	75	9	½	4	2	1.0	7	1106	1
Chili beef, w/ beans	1 cup	170	21	1	7	7	3.5	13	1035	10
Chunky, Campbell's®										
beef, w/ vegetable	1 cup	150	14	1	10	4	1.0	25	900	1
beef pasta	1 cup	150	18	1	13	3	1.0	20	970	2
cheese tortellini	1 cup	110	18	1	5	2	1.0	15	860	2
chicken, w/ wild rice	1 cup	140	18	1	9	3	1.0	25	840	2
chicken noodle	1 cup	130	16	1	9	3	1.0	20	1050	2
chicken vegetable	1 cup	165	19	1	12	5	1.0	17	1068	2
sirloin burger	1 cup	210	18	1	13	9	4.0	25	1010	4

SOUPS
Canned, prepared

ITEM	AMOUNT	CALORIES	CARBOHYDRATE (g)	CARBOHYDRATE CHOICES	PROTEIN (g)	FAT (g)	SATURATED FAT (g)	CHOLESTEROL (mg)	SODIUM (mg)	FIBER (g)
Chunky, Campbell's® *(con't.)*										
tomato ravioli	1 cup	150	26	2	5	3	1.5	10	970	3
vegetable	1 cup	130	22	1½	3	4	1.0	0	870	4
Clam chowder										
Manhattan	1 cup	78	12	1	2	2	0.0	2	578	1
New England*	1 cup	151	21	1½	8	4	2.0	5	1042	1
Corn chowder*	1 cup	141	24	1½	5	3	1.0	5	662	2
Cream of asparagus*	1 cup	161	15	1	7	8	3.0	5	972	1
Cream of broccoli*	1 cup	151	15	1	6	7	3.5	5	832	1
Cream of celery	1 cup	110	9	½	2	7	2.5	0	900	1
Cream of mushroom										
condensed, lowfat	½ cup	70	9	½	1	3	1.0	0	830	0
condensed, regular	½ cup	110	9	½	2	7	2.5	0	870	1
low sodium, ready to serve	1 cup	152	14	1	2	11	3.0	15	50	2
lowfat*	1 cup	70	9	½	1	3	1.0	5	830	1
regular*	1 cup	203	15	1	6	14	5.0	20	1076	1
Cream of potato*	1 cup	141	20	1	6	4	2.5	15	952	1
Cream of shrimp*	1 cup	151	14	1	6	8	3.0	25	952	1
Double Noodle®	1 cup	100	15	1	4	2.5	1.0	15	810	2
Escarole	1 cup	25	3	0	1	1	0.0	0	930	1
French onion	1 cup	57	8	½	2	2	0.0	1	902	0
Gazpacho	1 cup	56	1	0	9	2	1.0	0	1183	4
Green pea	1 cup	180	29	1½	9	3	1.0	0	890	5
Healthy Choice®										
broccoli & cheddar	1 cup	90	18	1	2	2	1.0	0	480	2
chicken Alfredo	1 cup	120	18	1	9	2	1.0	10	480	0
chicken noodle	1 cup	120	18	1	8	3	1.0	10	480	2
chili beef	1 cup	160	29	1½	16	2	0.5	10	440	7
creamy potato & ham	1 cup	120	19	1	7	2	1.0	5	480	2
garden vegetable	1 cup	110	23	1½	5	1	0.0	0	480	2
minestrone	1 cup	110	22	1	5	1	0.5	0	480	6
split pea & ham	1 cup	150	25	1½	12	2	0.5	0	480	3
Hot & sour	1 cup	133	5	0	12	6	2.0	23	1563	0
Lentil	1 cup	140	22	1	9	2	0.0	0	750	7
Lobster bisque*	1 cup	111	14	1	5	3	1.0	5	832	0
Matzo ball	1 cup	40	9	½	1	1	0.5	0	1290	1
Minestrone	1 cup	82	11	1	4	3	1.0	2	911	1
Mushroom	1 cup	80	10	½	2	3	1.0	0	930	1
Oyster stew*	1 cup	121	17	1	6	4	2.5	15	742	0
Pasta e fagioli	1 cup	194	30	2	9	5	1.0	3	790	2
Pepperpot	1 cup	100	9	½	4	5	2.0	15	1020	1
Ratatouille	1 cup	266	12	1	2	25	3.0	0	329	1

SOUPS
Canned, prepared

ITEM	AMOUNT	CALORIES	CARBOHYDRATE (g)	CARBOHYDRATE CHOICES	PROTEIN (g)	FAT (g)	SATURATED FAT (g)	CHOLESTEROL (mg)	SODIUM (mg)	FIBER (g)
Scotch broth	1 cup	80	9	½	4	3	1.5	10	870	1
Seafood chowder*	1 cup	131	15	1	11	3	1.0	20	692	0
Split pea, w/ ham	1 cup	190	28	1½	10	4	2.0	8	1007	5
Tomato										
bisque*	1 cup	174	29	2	6	4	1.5	11	1109	1
creamy, ready to serve	1 cup	100	22	1½	2	1	0.0	0	790	1
regular, w/ milk*	1 cup	131	24	1½	6	1	1.0	5	791	0
regular, w/ water	1 cup	85	17	1	2	1	0.0	0	871	0
w/ rice, ready to serve	1 cup	120	23	1½	2	2	0.5	0	790	1
Turkey noodle	1 cup	68	9	½	4	2	1.0	5	815	1
Vegetable	1 cup	72	12	1	2	2	0.0	0	821	0
Vegetable beef	1 cup	78	10	½	6	2	1.0	5	791	1
Vegetable broth	1 cup	20	3	0	2	1	0.0	0	1000	0
Vegetarian vegetable	1 cup	90	18	1	3	1	0.0	0	770	2
Wild rice, w/ chicken	1 cup	100	15	1	6	2	1.0	20	820	2
Dehydrated & Prepared, unless indicated										
Beef noodle	1 cup	40	6	½	2	1	0.0	3	1042	1
Bouillon, dry										
beef	1 cube	5	0	0	0	0	0.0	0	900	0
chicken	1 cube	5	0	0	0	0	0.0	0	1100	0
vegetable	1 cube	5	0	0	0	0	0.0	0	980	0
Chicken noodle	1 cup	53	7	½	3	1	0.0	3	1283	1
Chicken rice	1 cup	61	9	½	2	1	0.0	3	982	1
Cream of vegetable	1 cup	100	12	1	2	5	1.5	0	870	1
Cup Noodles®										
beef	1 (14 oz.)	300	38	2½	6	14	7.0	0	1080	2
chicken	1 (14 oz.)	300	36	2½	6	14	7.0	0	1170	2
Cup-a-Soup®										
chicken noodle	1 (6 oz.)	50	8	½	2	1	0.0	10	540	0
hearty chicken noodle	1 (6 oz.)	60	10	½	3	1	0.0	15	590	0
tomato	1 (6 oz.)	90	20	1	2	1	0.0	5	510	0
Leek	1 cup	71	19	1	2	2	1.0	3	965	3
Minestrone	1 cup	100	18	1	2	2	1.0	0	810	3
Mushroom	1 cup	96	11	1	2	5	1.0	0	1020	1
Onion	1 cup	27	5	0	1	1	0.0	0	849	1
Onion soup mix, dry	2 T.	45	8	½	1	1	0.5	0	790	0
Ramen noodle	1 cup	190	26	2	4	8	4.0	0	900	1
Tomato	1 cup	103	19	1	2	2	1.0	0	943	1
Vegetable beef	1 cup	53	8	½	3	1	1.0	0	1002	1

* Prepared w/ ½ cup 1% milk. If prepared w/ whole
milk add 24 calories, 3 g fat and 12 mg cholesterol.
If prepared w/ skim milk subtract 8 calories and 1 g fat.

VEGETABLES

ITEM	AMOUNT	CALORIES	CARBOHYDRATE (g)	CARBOHYDRATE CHOICES	PROTEIN (g)	FAT (g)	SATURATED FAT (g)	CHOLESTEROL (mg)	SODIUM (mg)	FIBER (g)
VEGETABLES										
Alfalfa sprouts, raw	½ cup	5	1	0	1	0	0.0	0	1	0
Artichokes										
boiled/steamed	1 medium	60	13	½	4	0	0.0	0	114	6
hearts, marinated	½ cup	112	9	0	3	9	1.0	0	600	5
Asparagus, cooked	½ cup	22	4	0	2	0	0.0	0	10	1
Bamboo shoots, raw	½ cup	20	4	0	2	0	0.0	0	3	2
Bean sprouts, raw	½ cup	16	3	0	2	0	0.0	0	3	1
Beets, pickled	½ cup	74	19	1	1	0	0.0	0	300	2
Bok choy, cooked	½ cup	10	2	0	1	0	0.0	0	29	1
Broccoli										
cooked	½ cup	22	4	0	2	0	0.0	0	20	2
cooked, w/ cheese sauce	½ cup	110	6	½	6	7	3.5	15	365	2
raw	½ cup	12	2	0	1	0	0.0	0	12	1
Brussel sprouts, cooked	½ cup	30	7	½	2	0	0.0	0	16	2
Cabbage										
Chinese, cooked	½ cup	11	2	0	1	0	0.0	0	55	1
green, cooked	½ cup	17	3	0	1	0	0.0	0	6	2
red, raw	½ cup	9	2	0	1	0	0.0	0	4	1
Carrots										
cooked	½ cup	35	8	½	1	0	0.0	0	51	2
raw	1 large	31	7	½	1	0	0.0	0	25	2
Cauliflower										
cooked	½ cup	14	3	0	1	0	0.0	0	9	1
raw	½ cup	13	3	0	1	0	0.0	0	15	1
w/ cheese sauce, cooked	½ cup	73	5	0	3	5	2.0	10	258	1
Celery										
cooked	½ cup	12	3	0	1	0	0.0	0	65	1
raw	1 stalk	6	1	0	0	0	0.0	0	35	1
Chinese-style, frzn.	½ cup	44	9	½	3	0	0.0	0	302	3
Chives, raw	1 T.	1	0	0	0	0	0.0	0	0	0
Corn, cooked										
cream-style, can	½ cup	92	23	1½	2	1	0.0	0	365	2
on the cob	1 medium	123	30	2	4	1	0.0	0	6	3
w/ butter sauce, frzn.	½ cup	115	23	1½	3	3	1.5	5	216	2
whole kernel, can	½ cup	66	15	1	2	1	0.0	0	175	2
whole kernel, frzn.	½ cup	66	16	1	2	0	0.0	0	4	2
Cucumbers, raw										
w/ skin	½ medium	20	4	0	1	0	0.0	0	3	1
w/o skin	½ cup	7	1	0	0	0	0.0	0	1	0
Eggplant, cooked	½ cup	14	3	0	0	0	0.0	0	1	1
Endive, raw	1 cup	9	2	0	1	0	0.0	0	11	2

VEGETABLES

ITEM	AMOUNT	CALORIES	CARBOHYDRATE (g)	CARBOHYDRATE CHOICES	PROTEIN (g)	FAT (g)	SATURATED FAT (g)	CHOLESTEROL (mg)	SODIUM (mg)	FIBER (g)
Green beans, cooked										
French style	½ cup	25	6	½	1	0	0.0	0	3	2
snap	½ cup	22	5	0	1	0	0.0	0	2	2
Green onions, raw	¼ cup	8	2	0	0	0	0.0	0	4	1
Greens, cooked										
beet	½ cup	19	4	0	2	0	0.0	0	174	2
collard	½ cup	25	5	0	2	0	0.0	0	9	3
dandelion	½ cup	17	3	0	1	0	0.0	0	23	2
mustard	½ cup	11	1	0	2	0	0.0	0	11	1
turnip	½ cup	14	3	0	1	0	0.0	0	21	3
Hominy, cooked	½ cup	58	11	1	1	1	0.0	0	168	2
Italian-style, frzn.	½ cup	48	5	0	1	3	1.0	5	130	1
Jicama, cooked/raw	½ cup	23	5	0	1	0	0.0	0	2	3
Kale, cooked	½ cup	18	4	0	1	0	0.0	0	15	1
Kohlrabi, cooked	½ cup	24	6	½	1	0	0.0	0	17	1
Leeks, raw	¼ cup	14	3	0	0	0	0.0	0	4	0
Lettuce, raw	1 cup	7	1	0	1	0	0.0	0	5	1
Mixed, frzn.	½ cup	54	12	1	3	0	0.0	0	32	4
Mushrooms										
can	½ cup	20	2	0	2	0	0.0	0	448	1
fried	5 medium	148	8	½	2	12	2.0	14	121	1
raw	½ cup	9	2	0	1	0	0.0	0	1	0
Okra, cooked	½ cup	26	6	½	2	0	0.0	0	4	2
Onions										
can	½ cup	21	4	0	1	0	0.0	0	416	1
chopped, raw	½ cup	30	7	½	1	0	0.0	0	2	1
rings, breaded & fried	5	164	21	1½	2	9	2.0	0	321	1
Parsley, raw	¼ cup	5	1	0	0	0	0.0	0	8	1
Parsnips, cooked	½ cup	63	15	1	1	0	0.0	0	8	3
Pea pods, cooked	½ cup	34	6	½	3	0	0.0	0	3	2
Peas, green, cooked	½ cup	67	12	1	4	0	0.0	0	2	4
Peppers, raw										
bell, green/red/yellow	½ cup	20	5	0	1	0	0.0	0	1	1
chiles, green, diced	¼ cup	15	3	0	1	0	0.0	0	30	0
jalapeños	1	11	2	0	0	0	0.0	0	2	0
Pimentos, can	¼ cup	11	2	0	1	0	0.0	0	7	1
Potatoes, cooked										
au gratin, box	½ cup	150	22	1½	2	6	1.5	0	630	1
baked, w/ skin	1 (4 oz.)	124	29	2	3	0	0.0	0	9	3
blintzes, frzn.	1 (2.3 oz.)	90	15	1	3	4	1.0	5	170	2
boiled, w/o skin	1 (4 oz.)	98	23	1½	2	0	0.0	0	6	2
French fries, frzn.	10 medium	100	16	1	2	4	1.0	0	15	2

VEGETABLES

ITEM	AMOUNT	CALORIES	CARBOHYDRATE (g)	CARBOHYDRATE CHOICES	PROTEIN (g)	FAT (g)	SATURATED FAT (g)	CHOLESTEROL (mg)	SODIUM (mg)	FIBER (g)
Potatoes, cooked *(con't.)*										
hash browns, frzn.	½ cup	160	14	1	1	11	3.0	0	310	1
instant, w/ marg. & milk	½ cup	160	19	1	3	8	1.5	5	460	1
knish, frzn.	1 (2 oz.)	201	20	1	4	11	2.0	54	219	1
mashed, w/ marg. & milk	½ cup	111	18	1	2	4	1.0	2	310	2
O'Brien, frzn.	½ cup	198	21	1½	2	13	3.0	0	42	2
pancakes, hmde.	1 medium	207	22	1½	5	12	2.0	73	386	2
pierogies, frzn.	3 (1.4 oz.)	180	34	2	6	2	0.0	0	340	2
scalloped, box	½ cup	160	21	1½	2	6	1.5	0	610	1
scalloped, w/ ham, hmde.	½ cup	117	13	1	6	5	3.0	19	539	1
Tater Tots®, frzn.	9	150	20	1	2	8	1.5	0	290	2
twice baked, w/ cheese	1 (5 oz.)	194	28	2	4	8	2.5	0	470	3
Pumpkin, can	½ cup	42	10	½	1	0	0.0	0	6	3
Radishes, raw	10	9	2	0	0	0	0.0	0	11	1
Rutabagas, cooked	½ cup	47	11	1	2	0	0.0	0	24	2
Salad greens, raw	1 cup	9	2	0	1	0	0.0	0	14	1
Sauerkraut, can	½ cup	22	5	0	1	0	0.0	0	780	3
Scallions, raw	1 T.	2	0	0	0	0	0.0	0	1	0
Shallots, raw	¼ cup	29	7	½	1	0	0.0	0	5	0
Spinach										
cooked	½ cup	21	3	0	3	0	0.0	0	63	2
creamed	½ cup	84	10	½	4	3	1.5	0	524	2
raw	1 cup	12	2	0	2	0	0.0	0	44	2
Squash										
acorn, cooked	½ cup	57	15	½	1	0	0.0	0	4	5
butternut, cooked	½ cup	47	12	1	1	0	0.0	0	2	3
summer, cooked/raw	½ cup	18	4	0	1	0	0.0	0	1	1
winter, cooked	½ cup	47	11	1	1	1	0.0	0	1	3
zucchini, cooked	½ cup	14	4	0	1	0	0.0	0	3	1
zucchini, raw	½ cup	9	2	0	1	0	0.0	0	2	1
Succotash, cooked	½ cup	110	23	1½	5	1	0.0	0	16	4
Sweet potatoes										
baked	1 (4 oz.)	117	28	2	2	0	0.0	0	11	3
candied, can	½ cup	240	60	4	1	0	0.0	0	15	2
mashed, w/o fat	½ cup	172	40	2½	3	0	0.0	0	21	3
Swiss chard, cooked	½ cup	18	4	0	2	0	0.0	0	157	2
Tomatoes										
cherry, raw	6 medium	21	5	0	1	0	0.0	0	9	1
paste, can	½ cup	120	24	1½	8	0	0.0	0	81	4
puree, can	½ cup	50	12	1	2	0	0.0	0	499	3
stewed, can	½ cup	43	9	½	1	0	0.0	0	252	1
sun dried	½ cup	70	15	1	4	0	0.0	0	566	3

VEGETABLES

ITEM	AMOUNT	CALORIES	CARBOHYDRATE (g)	CARBOHYDRATE CHOICES	PROTEIN (g)	FAT (g)	SATURATED FAT (g)	CHOLESTEROL (mg)	SODIUM (mg)	FIBER (g)
Tomatoes *(con't.)*										
whole, can	½ cup	23	5	0	1	0	0.0	0	178	1
whole, raw	1 medium	26	6	½	1	0	0.0	0	11	1
Turnips, cooked	½ cup	24	6	½	1	0	0.0	0	58	2
Water chestnuts, can	½ cup	35	9	½	1	0	0.0	0	6	2
Watercress, raw	½ cup	2	0	0	0	0	0.0	0	7	0
Wax beans, cooked	½ cup	22	5	0	1	0	0.0	0	2	1
Yams, baked/boiled	½ cup	79	19	1	1	0	0.0	0	5	3

For dried beans, peas and lentils see
Vegetarian Foods & Legumes.

VEGETARIAN FOODS & LEGUMES

Cooked w/o salt unless indicated

ITEM	AMOUNT	CALORIES	CARBOHYDRATE (g)	CARBOHYDRATE CHOICES	PROTEIN (g)	FAT (g)	SATURATED FAT (g)	CHOLESTEROL (mg)	SODIUM (mg)	FIBER (g)
Aduki/adzuki beans										
dry, cooked	½ cup	147	29	1½	9	0	0.0	0	9	6
sweetened, can	½ cup	351	81	5½	6	0	0.0	0	323	4
Bac-O's®	1½ T.	30	2	0	3	2	0.0	0	120	0
Bacon, vegetarian	1 slice	16	0	0	1	1	0.0	0	73	0
Baked beans, can										
vegetarian	½ cup	118	26	1	6	1	0.0	0	504	6
w/ molasses	½ cup	190	27	1	7	7	2.0	6	532	7
Black beans										
can	½ cup	100	17	½	7	1	0.0	0	400	7
dry, cooked	½ cup	114	20	1	8	0	0.0	0	1	7
Black eyed peas/cowpeas										
can	½ cup	120	21	1	7	1	0.0	0	350	6
dry, cooked	½ cup	80	17	1	3	0	0.0	0	3	4
Black turtle beans										
can	½ cup	109	20	1	7	0	0.0	0	461	8
dry, cooked	½ cup	120	23	1	8	0	0.0	0	3	5
Brewer's yeast	2 T.	106	9	½	15	0	0.0	0	36	0
Broad/fava beans										
can	½ cup	110	20	1	6	1	0.0	0	250	5
dry, cooked	½ cup	94	17	1	6	0	0.0	0	4	5
Burgers, vegetarian, frzn.										
Bocaburger®	1 (2.5 oz.)	84	9	0	12	0	0.0	0	338	5
Chik Patties®	1 (2.5 oz.)	150	15	1	9	6	1.0	0	570	2
Gardenburger®, original	1 (2.5 oz.)	130	18	1	8	3	1.0	10	290	5
Butter beans										
can	½ cup	90	16	1	6	0	0.0	0	453	4
frozen	½ cup	100	20	1	6	0	0.0	0	130	4
Calico beans, can	½ cup	126	24	1	8	0	0.0	0	240	9

VEGETARIAN FOODS & LEGUMES

ITEM	AMOUNT	CALORIES	CARBOHYDRATE (g)	CARBOHYDRATE CHOICES	PROTEIN (g)	FAT (g)	SATURATED FAT (g)	CHOLESTEROL (mg)	SODIUM (mg)	FIBER (g)
Cannellini beans, can	½ cup	100	18	1	5	1	0.0	0	270	5
Chickpeas/garbanzo beans										
can	½ cup	143	27	1½	6	1	0.0	0	359	5
dry, cooked	½ cup	134	22	1½	7	2	0.0	0	6	4
Chik Nuggets™, frzn.	4	160	17	1	13	4	0.5	0	670	5
Chili, vegetarian, can										
no added salt	1 cup	160	28	1	13	1	0.0	0	65	12
regular	1 cup	200	38	2	12	1	0.0	0	780	7
Chili beans, can	½ cup	110	24	1	7	1	0.5	0	360	7
Cranberry beans										
can	½ cup	108	20	1	7	0	0.0	0	432	8
dry, cooked	½ cup	120	22	1	8	0	0.0	0	1	9
Crowder peas, frzn.	½ cup	120	22	1½	8	1	0.0	0	10	4
Falafel patties	1 (0.6 oz.)	57	5	0	2	3	0.5	0	50	1
Great northern beans										
can	½ cup	70	17	1	6	0	0.0	0	490	6
dry, cooked	½ cup	104	19	1	7	0	0.0	0	2	6
Ground meat alternative	½ cup	70	5	0	12	0	0.0	0	200	3
Hot dogs										
tofu	1 (1.5 oz.)	60	2	0	8	3	1.0	0	140	0
veggie	1 (2 oz.)	80	6	½	11	1	0.0	0	580	1
Hummus	½ cup	210	25	1	6	10	1.5	0	300	6
Kidney beans										
can	½ cup	104	19	1	7	0	0.0	0	444	4
dry, cooked	½ cup	112	20	1	8	0	0.0	0	2	6
Lentils, cooked	½ cup	115	20	1	9	0	0.0	0	2	9
Lima beans										
baby, frzn.	½ cup	95	18	1	6	0	0.0	0	26	5
can	½ cup	95	18	1	6	0	0.0	0	405	6
dry, cooked	½ cup	108	20	1	7	0	0.0	0	2	7
Miso	2 T.	71	10	½	4	2	0.5	0	1254	2
Mung beans, dry, cooked	½ cup	106	19	1	7	0	0.0	0	2	8
Natto	½ cup	186	13	½	16	10	1.5	0	6	5
Navy beans										
can	½ cup	148	27	1	10	1	0.0	0	587	7
dry, cooked	½ cup	129	24	1	8	1	0.0	0	1	6
Pigeonpeas, dry, cooked	½ cup	102	20	1	6	0	0.0	0	4	6
Pink beans, dry, cooked	½ cup	126	24	1½	8	0	0.0	0	2	4
Pinto beans										
can	½ cup	103	18	1	6	1	0.0	0	353	6
dry, cooked	½ cup	117	22	1	7	0	0.0	0	2	7
Red beans	½ cup	121	23	1	7	0	0.0	0	231	9

VEGETARIAN FOODS & LEGUMES

ITEM	AMOUNT	CALORIES	CARBOHYDRATE (g)	CARBOHYDRATE CHOICES	PROTEIN (g)	FAT (g)	SATURATED FAT (g)	CHOLESTEROL (mg)	SODIUM (mg)	FIBER (g)
Refried beans, can										
fat free	½ cup	110	20	1	7	0	0.0	0	530	8
regular	½ cup	140	23	1	8	3	0.5	0	480	6
Sandwich slices, vegetarian	2	90	8	½	14	0	0.0	0	270	1
Sausages, vegetarian, frzn.										
links	1 (1 oz.)	64	2	0	5	5	1.0	0	222	1
patties	1 (1.5 oz.)	109	4	0	8	8	1.5	0	378	1
Seitan, dry	½ cup	227	21	1½	32	2	0.0	0	30	3
Soy meal, defatted	½ cup	206	22	1	30	1	0.0	0	2	11
Soy protein										
concentrate	1 oz.	94	9	½	16	0	0.0	0	1	2
isolate	1 oz.	96	2	0	23	1	0.0	0	285	2
Soybeans										
dry roasted, salted	¼ cup	127	9	0	10	7	1.0	0	164	8
green, cooked	½ cup	127	10	½	11	6	0.5	0	13	4
mature, cooked	½ cup	149	9	0	15	8	1.0	0	1	5
organic, can	½ cup	150	11	1	13	7	1.0	0	140	3
Split peas, dry, cooked	½ cup	116	21	1	8	0	0.0	0	2	8
Stakelets®, frzn.	1 (2.5 oz.)	140	6	½	12	8	1.0	0	480	2
Tempeh	½ cup	165	14	1	16	6	1.0	0	5	4
Tofu										
firm	3 oz.	60	2	0	6	3	0.0	0	10	0
flavored, baked	3 oz.	180	5	0	20	9	1.5	0	360	1
soft	3 oz.	45	1	0	5	3	0.0	0	15	0
White beans, dry, cooked	½ cup	124	23	1	9	0	0.0	0	5	6

Favorite Foods

ITEM	AMOUNT	CALORIES	CARBOHYDRATE (g)	CARBOHYDRATE CHOICES	PROTEIN (g)	FAT (g)	SATURATED FAT (g)	CHOLESTEROL (mg)	SODIUM (mg)	FIBER (g)
Corn Chowder	1/5	311	29		9	14 (40%)				2
Easiest Waffles	1	512	56		8.6	29 (51%)				2.2
" " w/ unsweetened applesauce	1	442	57		8.6	20.3 (42%)				1
Waffles w/ applesauce	1/2	221	28.5		4.3	10	"			.5
Smores (1 sheet)		143	26		1	4.5 (27%)				.5
" 1/2		72	13		.5	2.3				.3
Rootbeer float w/ diet Rawgr & Lowfat froz. vanilla yogurt		90	17		3	1.5 (15%)				0

Favorite Foods

ITEM	AMOUNT	CALORIES	CARBOHYDRATE (g)	CARBOHYDRATE CHOICES	PROTEIN (g)	FAT (g)	SATURATED FAT (g)	CHOLESTEROL (mg)	SODIUM (mg)	FIBER (g)

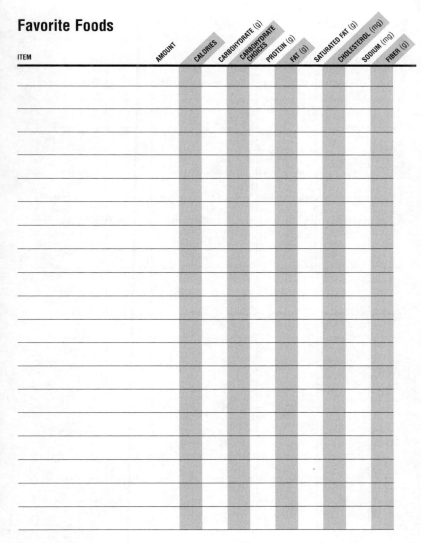

Know Your Numbers

Date	Cholesterol	LDL	HDL	Triglycerides	Blood Pressure	Weight	Other/Comments

Medications/Supplements

Start Date	Name of Medication & Dosage	Comments	Stop Date

Desirable Levels:
Blood Lipids & Blood Pressure

	General Population	Diabetes	Coronary Heart Disease
Cholesterol	<200 mg/dl	<200 mg/dl	<180 mg/dl
LDL	<130 mg/dl	<130 mg/dl	<100 mg/dl
HDL	>35 mg/dl	>35 mg/dl	>55 mg/dl
Triglycerides	<200 mg/dl	<160 mg/dl	<200 mg/dl
Blood Pressure	<140/90 mg/dl	<135/85 mg/dl	<140/90 mg/dl

Goals

Cholesterol: _____

LDL: _____

HDL: _____

Triglycerides: _____

Blood Pressure: _____

Weight: _____

Food Guide Pyramid

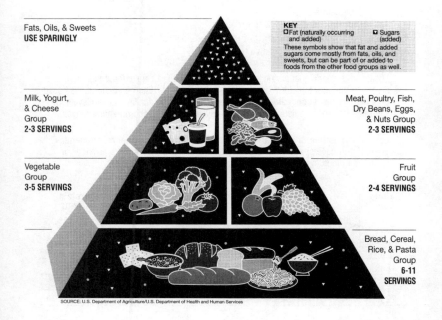

Fats, Oils, & Sweets
USE SPARINGLY

KEY
☐ Fat (naturally occurring and added)   ▨ Sugars (added)
These symbols show that fat and added sugars come mostly from fats, oils, and sweets, but can be part of or added to foods from the other food groups as well.

Milk, Yogurt, & Cheese Group
2-3 SERVINGS

Meat, Poultry, Fish, Dry Beans, Eggs, & Nuts Group
2-3 SERVINGS

Vegetable Group
3-5 SERVINGS

Fruit Group
2-4 SERVINGS

Bread, Cereal, Rice, & Pasta Group
6-11 SERVINGS

SOURCE: U.S. Department of Agriculture/U.S. Department of Health and Human Services

Estimate your Daily Nutrient Goals in Three Easy Steps

Step 1

Determine your recommended calorie goal using the information below. If you want to lose between one-half to one pound per week, subtract 250-500 calories from the recommended ranges. For a balanced diet, women should not eat less than 1200 calories and men should not eat less than 1500 calories each day.

1500-1800 calories
Sedentary women and some older adults

1800-2400 calories
Active women and many sedentary men

2400-2800 calories
Active men and some very active women

Step 2

Locate your calorie goal on the left-hand side of the chart below. Read the chart across to the right to determine your other nutrient goals. Each nutrient goal is based on a percentage of your calorie goal. Three different levels for fat and two levels for saturated fat goals are listed. Your goal is to eat within the recommended ranges.

Step 3

Look at the bottom of the chart for cholesterol, sodium and fiber recommendations. If you have special nutrient needs, talk with your health care provider or registered dietitian for the amounts that are right for you.

Calorie Goal	Fat Grams			Saturated Fat Grams		Carbohydrate Grams	Protein Grams
	30%	25%	20%	10%	7%	50-60%	10-15%
1200	40	33	27	13	9	150-180	30-45
1500	50	42	33	17	12	188-225	38-56
1800	60	50	40	20	14	225-270	45-68
2000	67	56	44	22	16	250-300	50-75
2200	73	61	49	24	17	275-330	55-83
2500	83	69	56	28	19	313-375	63-94
2800	93	78	62	31	22	350-420	70-105

Cholesterol	Sodium	Fiber
300 milligrams	2400 milligrams	25 to 35 grams

If you have diabetes and are counting carbohydrate grams or carbohydrate choices, each has been provided for you in this book. The amount of carbohydrate grams and choices you can eat is based on your calorie goal.

Carbohydrate Goals for Diabetes

Calorie Goal	Carbohydrate Grams	Carbohydrate Choices
1200	150-180	10-12
1500	188-225	13-15
1800	225-270	15-18
2000	250-300	17-20
2200	275-330	18-22
2500	313-375	21-25
2800	350-420	23-28

Carbohydrate choices have been calculated using the 15-Gram Equation (15 grams of carbohydrate = 1 carbohydrate choice). We have done the calculating for you for all foods listed in this book. Since fiber is part of the total carbohydrate, when fiber was 5 grams or greater, it was subtracted from the total carbohydrate grams before calculating carbohydrate choices.

Carbohydrate Grams	Carbohydrate Choices
0-5	0
6-10	½
11-20	1
21-25	1½
26-35	2
36-40	2½
41-50	3
51-55	3½
56-65	4
66-70	4½
71-80	5

Looking for an Individualized Eating Plan?

A registered dietitian (RD) can help. To locate an RD in your area, contact The American Dietetic Association's referral service by calling 1-800-366-1655 or visit the website at www.eatright.org.

Calories Used Through Activity

Estimate the number of calories used during 30 minutes of various activities.

Activity	30 min.
Aerobic dance	210
Archery	132
Badminton	198
Baseball	141
Basketball	282
Bicycling	
6 mph	120
8 mph	156
10 mph	192
12 mph	261
Bowling	98
Boxing	282
Canoeing, 4 mph	90
Dancing	
fast	204
slow	144
Farming, light	81
Fencing	159
Fishing	126
Football	150
Gardening	144
Golfing	
cart	87
walk	162
Handball	294

Activity	30 min.
Hiking, 3 mph	204
Hockey	
field	273
ice	315
Horseback riding	225
Housework	132
Hunting	180
Ice skating	192
Jogging, 5 mph	273
Judo/karate	399
Jumping rope	330
Mountain climbing	324
Mowing lawn, manual	110
Painting, outside	156
Pool (billiards)	66
Racquetball	294
Roller blading	192
Roller skating	192
Rowing machine	243
Running	
8 mph	438
10 mph	546
Sailing	90
Scuba diving	390

Calories Used Through Activity *(con't.)*

Activity	30 min.	Activity	30 min.
Sitting	.57	Tennis	
Skiing		doubles	.156
downhill	.297	singles	.225
X-country, 4 mph	.297	Treading water	.126
Sleeping	.45	Treadmill, 4 mph	.198
Snow shoveling	.203	Volleyball	.102
Soccer	.279	Walking	
Softball	.141	3 mph	.150
Squash	.432	4 mph	.198
Stair climbing	.330	5 mph	.246
Standing, light work	.123	Water-Skiing	.225
Swimming		Weight training	.189
fast	.318	Wrestling	.396
slow	.261	Yoga	.126
Table tennis	.138		

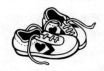

Calorie values are approximate and vary based on an individual's weight, exertion and skill level. Values were calculated for a 150-pound person. To adjust for your weight: divide your weight by 150, then multiply this number (your weight factor) by the calorie values on this chart.

References

Books and Periodicals

McArdle, William D., et al. "Energy Expenditure in Household, Occupational, Recreational, and Sports Activities." In *Exercise Physiology: Energy, Nutrition and Human Performance.* Baltimore: Williams & Wilkins, 1996.

Monk, Arlene. *Convenience Food Facts.* 4th ed. Minneapolis: IDC Publishing, 1997.

Pennington, Jean A.T. *Bowes & Church's Food Values of Portions Commonly Used.* 17th ed. Philadelphia: Lippincott-Raven, 1998.

Wheeler, Madelyn L., Marion Franz, Phyllis Barrier, et al. "Macronutrient and Energy Database for the 1995 Exchange Lists for Meal Planning: A Rationale for Clinical Practice Decisions," *Journal of the American Dietetic Association* 96 (1996): 1167-1171.

Williams, MH. "Calorie Expenditure for Various Physical Activities." In *Nutrition for Fitness and Sport.* 2nd ed. New York: Wm C Brown Publishers, 1995.

Other

-Fast food franchise nutrition information.

-The Food Processor. Nutrition & Fitness Software. Version 7.20. 1998, (ESHA Research) Salem, OR.

-Manufacturer's Nutrition Facts food labels.

-National Cholesterol Education Program (NCEP) Guidelines, 1993.

-United States Department of Agriculture. The Food Guide Pyramid. 1992.

Index

Ground,
  beef, 66
  pork, 67-68
  turkey, 74-75
Gyros, 77
Half & half, 58
Ham, 67-68, 75
Hamburger, 26, *see also* Fast Foods
Hardee's®, 46-47
Honey, 30, 39
Hot cocoa, 10
Hot dogs, 26, 68, 73, 75
Hummus, 88
Ice cream, 36-37
  sandwiches, 37
  toppings, 37
  novelties, 36-37
Italian dishes, 77
  see also Combination Foods
  dressing, 79
Italian/Mediterranean entrées, 77
Jam/jelly, 39
Ketchup, 27
KFC®, 47-48
Kidney beans, 88
Kiwifruit, 65
Lamb, all cuts, 67
Lasagna, 25
Legumes, 87-89,
  see also Beans
  lentils, 88
  tofu, 89
Lemon, 65
  juice, 63
  meringue pie, 38
Lemonade, 10
Lentils, 88
Lettuce, 85
Lima beans, 88
Lime, 65
Lobster, 61
Luncheon meats, 67-68
Macaroni, 72
  & cheese, 25

Manicotti, 25
Maple syrup, 39
Margarine, 58
Marmalade, 39
Marshmallow creme, 39
Marshmallows, 16, 38
Mayonnaise, 58
McDonald's®, 48-50
MEATS, 66-69, *see also*
  Combination Foods, Fast Foods,
  Poultry, Restaurant Favorites,
  Soups
  beef, 66-68
  game, 67
  lamb, 67
  pork, 67
  processed & luncheon meats,
  67-68
  specialty & organ meats, 69
Melons, 64-66
Mexican entrées, 77-78
Milk, all types, 69-71
MILK & YOGURT, 69-71,
  see also Cheese
Milk shake, 70
Millet, 73
Molasses, 30
Mousse, 38
Mozzarella cheese, 21
Muffins, all types, 12-13
Mushrooms, 75, 85
Mustard, 28
Nachos, 75
Navy beans, 88
Noodles, all types, 72
NUTS, SEEDS & PEANUT BUTTER,
  all types, 71-72
Oat bran, 17, 19
Oatmeal, 17
  cookies, 36
Oils, all types, 58-59
Olives, 28
Omelets, 40
Onions, 85

Orange, 65
  drinks, 11
  juice, 63
Organ meats, 69
Ostrich, 74
Pancake syrup, 39
Pancakes, 13-14, 24
Parmesan cheese, 21
Parmigiana, chicken/veal, 23, 77
Pasta, 72
  dishes, 77
  types, 72
PASTA, RICE & OTHER GRAINS,
  72-73, *see also* Combination
  Foods, Restaurant Favorites,
  Salads
Pasta sauce, 72
Pastries, 34-35
Peaches, 65
Peanuts, 16, 71
Peanut butter, 71
  & jelly sandwich, 26
  cookies, 36
Pears, 65
Peas, 85, 87-89
Pecans, 71
Pepperoni, 68
Peppers, 85
Pesto sauce, 28
Pheasant, 74
Phyllo dough, 30
Pickles, 28
Pies, 38, 76
  chocolate, 38, 76
  cream, 38
  crusts, 30
  fruit fillings, 30
  meat, 25-26
Pilaf, 72
Pine nuts, 71
Pineapple, 65
Pinto beans, 88
Pizza, 25,
  see also specific Fast Foods